eat
yourself
thin

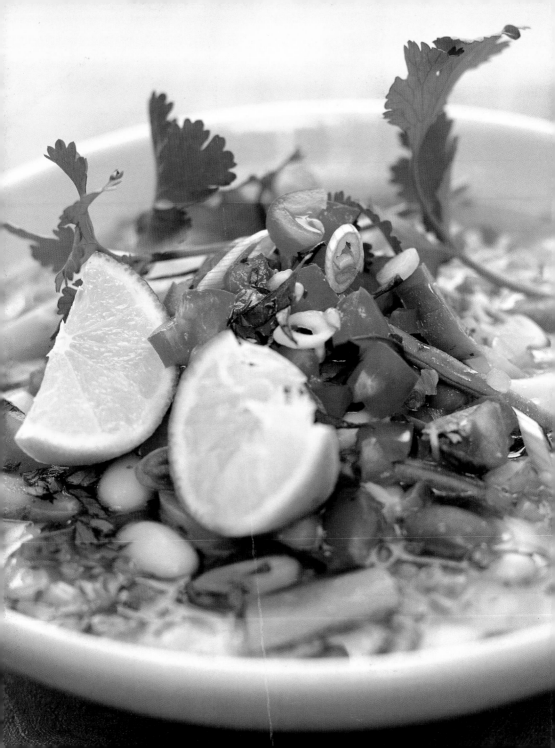

joanna hall

YOUR
ONE-STOP
GUIDE
TO HEALTHY
EATING AND
A FLATTER
TUMMY

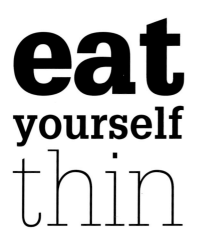

eat
yourself
thin

First published in Great Britain in 2008 by
Kyle Cathie Limited
122 Arlington Road, London NW1 7HP
www.kylecathie.com
The material in this book comes from Joanna Hall's *The Weight-Loss Bible*

10 9 8 7 6 5 4 3 2 1

ISBN 978-1-85626-835-6

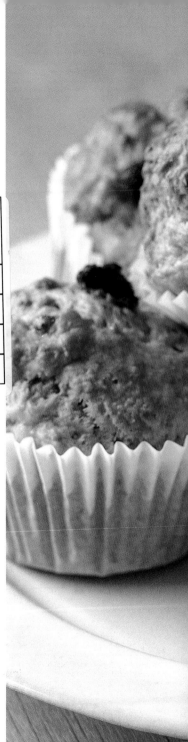

Text © 200
Book desig
Photograph
except pag
Alamy; 20 (
34/35 mood
StockFood.
39 (top) VV
42 eikonas

Joanna Hall is hereby identified as the author of this work in
accordance with Section 77 of the Copyright, Designs and
Patents Act 1988.

Project editor Vicki Murrell
Designer Abby Franklin
Photographer Dan Welldon
Recipes Louise Shaxson
Production Sha Huxtable

A Cataloguing In Publication record for this title is
available from the British Library.

Printed by TWP, Singapore

Contents

Introduction 6

1
So let's get to know you 8
- tell-tale signs of a fad diet ▪ your food IQ
- how many calories? ▪ the energy gap

2
What you eat 18
- a balanced diet ▪ the carb curfew
- healthy shopping ▪ the glycaemic index
- reading the label

3
How you eat 34
- how to cut calories in 7 easy steps
- the menu plans ▪ healthy eating for children

4
The recipes 46
- breakfasts ▪ lunches ▪ dinners
- puddings ▪ kid's food

Index 112

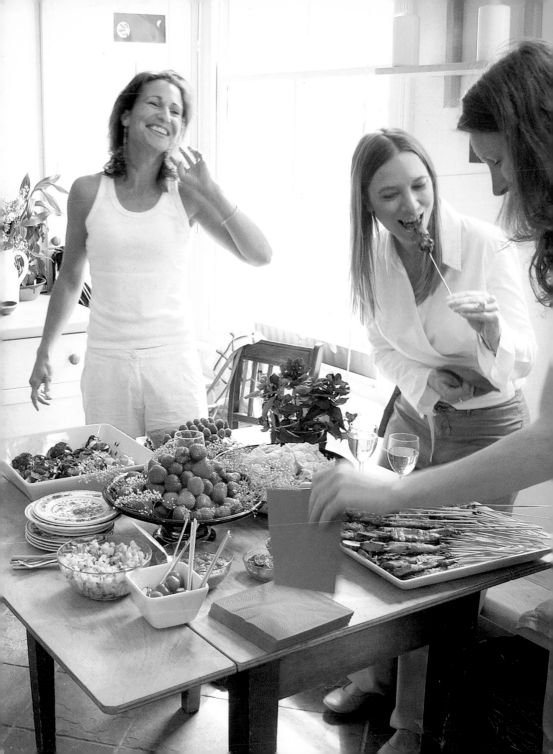

Introduction

Being successful with your weight-loss efforts doesn't mean you have to stop eating or say 'No' for the rest of your life to all those favourite foods that you love so much. Getting a better body is not just about the number of calories that pass your mouth, it's about being intelligent about your food and your physical activity. In *Eat yourself Thin* you'll learn how to eat smarter without the hassle of counting calories or feeling you have to put your life on hold.

In the '7 Ways to Cut Calories' section, I list the all-important principles for healthy eating so, if you always keep these in mind, you'll be armed with a set of tools that mean you can enjoy your food while also staving off the temptations. This will put you back in control for as soon as you understand why and how your body is susceptible to cravings and sugar highs, you can avoid the pitfalls that trip up all your good intentions.

Operating my Carb Curfew is one of the simplest and most effective strategies and means no pasta, rice, potatoes or bread after 5 pm. But don't worry as there are plenty of foods you can still enjoy as part of your evening meal – meat, fish, vegetables, essential fats and pulses – that, crucially, won't leave you feeling bloated or with a food hangover the next day. Give it a go and I guarantee you'll be surprised at how effective it can be.

And in the recipe section you'll find a delicious selection of my tried-and-tested, carb-curfew dishes; there are ideas for every occasion and each is clearly rated with the calorie and nutritional content of each meal so that you can pick and choose and plan ahead for the rest of the week.

And for the younger members of your family – check out the kid's food section to get them off to a flying start with mouthwatering recipes that give them the foods they love but with none of the hidden calories. Remember, the most important thing is for you to enjoy your food and feel confident that your eating choices will make a difference – eat yourself thin and you will transform the way you look and feel.

Be active

Joanna

So let's get to know you

Ditch the One-Night Stand!

Our eating habits play a fundamental part in the quality of our life and can provide us with a lot of pleasure as well as vital nutrients for good health. Quite simply, the condition of your body and the effectiveness of your training is directly related to the quality and quantity of the foods you consume and how well hydrated you are. So, with that in mind...ditch the one-night stand!

Successful weight loss is a lot like relationships. What we're looking for in a relationship – and what we're prepared to put into it – influence how it will turn out. Quick-fix diets are the one-night stands of the eating spectrum: in the same way as you realise that the night of passion with that person you fancied wasn't all you thought it would be, the 'revolutionary' new diet leaves you feeling exhausted, bad tempered and above all, disappointed.

Compare this with a long-term relationship. A good, lasting partnership involves a bit of work and upkeep. It's not always glamorous, and there are inevitably problems along the way, but you know it feels right, and ultimately it works long-term.

Over the years it will evolve, and it's the way in which you navigate the sometimes tricky road that determines the likelihood of long-term success. Your relationship with your body is exactly the same. So ditch that One-night Stand mentality now!

THE TELL-TALE SIGNS OF A FAD DIET

Fad diets tend to capture media attention, but they're the One-Night Stands of weight loss. At best, you'll regain the weight you've lost; at worst, you could damage your health. To become a fad-diet detective, look out for warning signs:

They often: promote magic or miracle foods, promise rapid weight loss, provide no exercise advice, stipulate bizarre quantities or specific food combinations, exclude entire food groups or prescribe rigid menus. You may recognise some of the following.

FOOD COMBINING

Claims: eating protein and carbohydrates in the same meal disrupts the digestion and produces toxins that make you fat; carbohydrates raise insulin levels, increase appetite and encourage fat storage, resulting in weight gain.

Reality check: The science aside, just ensuring you do not combine protein and carbohydrate in one meal is hard enough. For every meal, every day, it's next to impossible. Such a diet cannot be sustained in the long term. To make diets work, they have to fit in with your life.

HIGH-PROTEIN, LOW CARB

Claims: an excessive amount of insulin is released after you eat carbohydrate foods and this increases fat storage in the body. Often, in the first two weeks of a low-carb plan, you're allowed only 20g carbohydrate a day, so if you eat a banana (30g), you've blown it already. You progress to 40g carbs a day and then to the maintenance level of 60g. Consequently, these diets offer very limited food choices, while encouraging high protein and fat consumption. These diets also claim they dissolve fat tissue and thereby trigger more fat loss.

Reality check: No food is bad for your health when eaten in moderation. The World Health Organisation confirms the importance of carbs in the diet and research has shown that diets high in saturated fat can increase risks of obesity, cardiovascular disease and certain cancers. Ketosis, the bodily process resulting from excess protein intake and depletion of carbohydrates, can suppress appetite, but the side-effects are nausea, dizziness and bad breath.

SUGARBUSTERS/SUGAR CRAVERS

Claims: eating high Glycaemic Index carbs increases insulin and promotes body fat storage and obesity; fluids drunk with meals inhibit digestion and encourage fat storage. Some of these diets try to eliminate all carbs, so that calories are only obtained from protein and fat, and you are only allowed a very low calorie intake.

Reality check: Weight loss results from calorie reduction, not a decrease in insulin levels. There is no scientific evidence that fluids drunk with meals inhibit digestion.

THE ZONE

Claims: each meal should be composed of an optimum nutrient mix of 30 per cent fat, 30 per cent protein and 40 per cent carbs. This is the body's 'Zone', where body and mind are united for optimum performance and optimum weight loss.

Reality check: This 'macronutrient block method' has very little flexibility and views food purely as a drug.

NEVER SAY 'NO'

Nearly all foods can be fair game. Even when you're trying to restrict calories, indulging in a favourite treat is okay as long as portion sizes are controlled and it does not become a regular luxury.

Likewise, don't develop a phobia for a food, food group or component of food. Avoiding carbohydrates, fruits, sugars, protein or fat – whatever the fad diet of the moment may be – is a bad idea; instead, moderation is the key.

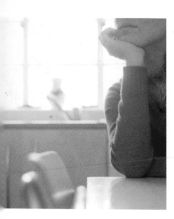

So just how good is your food IQ?

You think you know you're eating healthily – you're counting calories and stocking up on fruit and vegetables – but are you? Do the food IQ to see if the decisions you make as you navigate your day are the best ones to boost your health and energy.

1) Immediately you wake up, you need a quick drink to bring you round. There isn't time for breakfast, so what do you choose?
a) Water
b) Lashings of hot tea
c) A glass of diluted orange juice

2) Your weekday breakfast usually consists of:
a) Toast with butter and marmalade
b) A snatched Mars bar from a vending kiosk at the railway station
c) Muesli with yoghurt and some dried fruit

3) Mid-morning, you usually grab a drink of:
a) Coffee or tea, followed by water
b) Fresh juice, and plenty of it, diluted if necessary
c) Water

4) For lunch, which would you choose?

a) An egg-white omelette and some fresh fruit
b) A fast-food takeaway
c) A grilled chicken sandwich, packet of low-fat crisps and a banana

5) During the day, you:
a) Combat thirst when necessary by downing a lot of mineral water
b) Limit yourself to 4 cups of tea and coffee, and then drink diet, caffeine-free sodas
c) Sip water almost constantly, even when you don't feel thirsty

6) What is your daily pattern?
a) Eat three substantial meals a day, and try to avoid snacking
b) Eat less earlier in the day – because it's harder to resist naughty treats and snacks as the day wears on
c) Eat 4 or 5 times a day – but keep the portion sizes smaller and well-balanced

7) Before a visit to the gym, you:
   a) Eat and drink lightly, to avoid exercising on a full stomach
   b) Eat a good lunch, to give your body plenty of energy
   c) Don't eat – save your appetite until afterwards

8) After your workout, you:
   a) Wait for half an hour, and then eat a light snack
   b) Eat a banana immediately to restore energy levels
   c) Take advantage of your revved-up metabolism and avoid eating, so you can burn off more fat

9) In the pub, what best describes your drinking and eating habits?
   a) You choose 'long' drinks like wine spritzers or lagers, and avoid nibbling on crisps
   b) You drink whatever you like, but choose low-calorie mixers or colas to make up for the nuts you've munched
   c) You Drink wine or beer, but always have a glass of water in between each round.

10) Last thing at night – what do you do?
   a) Make sure you're full so you won't wake up hungry in the night
   b) Avoid eating at all – sleep on an empty stomach
   c) Eat some fresh fruit or raw vegetables, but make sure it's at least an hour before you go to sleep

HOW DID YOU SCORE?

Give yourself one point for every B answer, two points for every A answer, and 3 points for every C answer. If you scored:

10–16 POINTS

Your food IQ could use a good boost – and your body could well benefit from it too! It is not always easy to fit good nutrition into a busy life, so read through the answers on the following page that will help you get the most out of your nutrition.

17–23 POINTS

Your knowledge and food sense is pretty good, but the challenge often comes when you try to fit your knowledge into a busy life. So you should find all the tips on the following page really helpful – and with prior planning, you'll benefit from more energy too.

24–30 POINTS

You know your food facts, which means you are giving your body the best chance of an active and healthy life. Keep going, and the results will show for themselves.

Answers

1
a) Although water is good for hydrating the body, it won't add any vitamins or minerals to your diet.
b) One cup of tea can be good for a quick pick-me-up, but it acts as a diuretic and will make you urinate more frequently.
c) The best choice is diluted fruit juice as by diluting the concentrated juice you are helping to hydrate the body and to speed up the passage of nutrients crossing the stomach lining into the body.

2
a) Bread products have a high glycaemic index, which means they fill us up and then leave us feeling hungry as blood sugar levels fall.
b) A dose of highly refined sugar soon leaves you with a sugar 'slump', potentially leading to even more unhealthy snacking.
c) Muesli contains a good balance of nutrients and low to moderate glycaemic index carbohydrates, which release energy slowly right through the morning to fuel your body and your brain.

3
a) There's nothing wrong with a cup of coffee or tea, provided you compensate for the dehydrating effects by drinking plenty of water.
b) Fresh juices can be high in natural sugars and so are best diluted, plus watch out for all the hidden calories they can contain.
c) Water hydrates you and can reduce your 'sugar' cravings.

4
a) Egg-white omelettes and fruit may not give you all the calories and certainly not all the fat your body may need.
b) Fast food can be very high in unhealthy saturated fat, refined sugars and refined carbohydrates – best left for emergencies only.
c) A tasty sandwich, low-fat crisps and fruit will give your body all it needs to sustain you through the working day.

5
a) By the time you feel thirsty, your body is already dehydrated.
b) Even though some sodas may be caffeine- and sugar-free, they don't add any nutritional value, and are better replaced by water.
c) Sipping little and often also provides the best opportunity for your body to hydrate itself effectively. Even your skin will benefit.

eat yourself thin

6

a) A little protein with some source of starch at lunchtime will aid concentration and energy levels through the afternoon.

b) A steady calorific intake can be a very successful eating strategy, especially if you suffer from lapses of energy.

c) If you're often tempted to snack later on in the day, eat a healthy snack earlier together with some water to hydrate you.

7

a) Drink a small cup of water about 30 minutes before you start training, and throughout your workout sip little and often.

b) Your digestive system needs a supply of blood in order to digest food, but when you exercise your muscles also demand blood in order to carry oxyen to the working muscles. This results in a stitch.

c) Try to avoid eating for up to 2 hours before a workout.

8

a) Your muscle cells can replenish the essential glycogen stores most effectively within the first 2 hours after exercise.

b) A ripe banana will give you a ready supply of simple sugars which can easily be converted into glycogen to help your body repair.

c) After a workout your muscles are starving for nutrients and you can build up more muscle tissue if you eat high-quality protein.

9

a) Make sure you have had your 2 litres of water before you start to party and hydrate as you go through the night.

b) Nuts and crisps are high in fat and salt which will only increase your thirst. Too much salt can cause raised blood pressure.

c) By drinking water between each alcoholic drink, you'll help to combat the effects of dehydration.

10

a) Some nutrition experts believe that eating too near bedtime can increase the chances of you storing the calories as fat.

b) A glass of milk or a light carbohydrate snack can stimulate feelings of calm through the release of specific brain transmitters.

c) If you are hungry, the best idea is to have a light fruit snack, which will not place heavy digestive demands on your body late at night.

WHAT IS A CALORIE?

Look at any food label and you will see the terms Kcals (kilocalories) or Kjoules (kilojoules). These are units of energy. 'Calorie' is the most widely used term while 'kilojoule' is more often used in research. We'll use calories here, but if you need to convert an energy value, remember 1 kilocalorie = 4.2 kilojoules.

SO... HOW MANY CALORIES DO YOU NEED?

This all depends on how active you are and how much energy you use up in one day. An effective way of finding out is by filling in a 24-hour activity chart and colouring each hour according to what you are doing during that time. If you do this every day over the course of a week, you can then see at a glance how active your lifestyle is. Additionally, it is useful to be able to measure your activity levels by wearing some sort of tracking device, and the simplest and easiest of these is a pedometer. At the end of each day you can record the number of steps you have accumulated on your 24-hour colour chart.

MIND THE ENERGY GAP

Ensure you are regularly expending more calories through physical activity than you are consuming in food. If you Mind the Energy Gap, your weight will look after itself.

24-HOUR ACTIVITY CHART

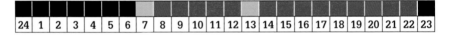

Think of your typical day as you colour in this chart
- Colour in black the time you are lying down
(sleeping, napping or stretched out on the sofa).
- Colour in pink all the time you are sitting
(at work, in a vehicle, at home; include such things as watching TV, reading, at a desk or computer, eating, and all sedentary leisure activities).
- Colour in orange the time you are on your feet (doing light activities in your day).
- Colour in yellow the time you are doing strength or resistance work
(include heavy manual lifting).
- Colour in green the time you are doing moderately intensephysical activity
(such as brisk walking).
- Colour in purple the time you are doing vigorous physical activity.

HOW DO YOU RATE?

Once you have filled in your 24-hour activity chart and established your average number of steps per day, have a look at the table below, drawn up from research conducted in Japan as a means of classifying activity levels.

If you are	Your activity factor is
Sedentary woman	12
Sedentary man	14
Active woman	15
Active man	17
Very active woman	18
Very active man	20

Under 5,000 steps a day — 'sedentary'
5,000–7,500 steps a day — 'low active'
7,500–10,000 steps a day — 'somewhat active'
10,000–12,500 steps a day — 'active'
12,500 steps a day + — 'highly active'

A simple way to calculate how many calories you need is to use the below table to find your activity factor. Multiply your activity factor by your current weight in pounds. The resulting number is the approximate number of calories you currently need to maintain your weight.

THE MATHS:

Activity factor x weight in pounds = current energy needs

For example, an active woman who weighs 150lb would need 2,250 calories a day (15 x 150 = 2,250).

If you want to achieve safe, effective weight loss, reduce your result by 500, and that will give you your new target. A reduction of 1,000 calories a day is achievable, but it will probably feel quite hard to maintain, so start with 500 calories – you can always cut back further once your new eating habits have evolved.

TO LOSE A POUND OF FAT

Losing a pound (0.45kg) of fat requires creating an Energy Gap of 3,500 calories. So if you want to lose 1lb in a week, that means reducing your intake by 500 calories each day. In theory, you could just eat small quantities of ice-cream and sweets and still lose weight, as long as your calorie intake is less than calories burnt. But before you leap for joy and head off to the corner shop, here's a word of warning: in the long term, choosing fruits, vegetables, whole grains and good sources of protein instead will not only facilitate weight management and prevent weight regain, but it will also ensure that you look and feel better. Choosing a diet that results in a permanent lifestyle change is essential for success. You will find the Menu Plans on pages 42–43 and Recipes in Chapter 4 very helpful for getting you on track. You'll soon realise that you can enjoy healthy foods just as much as the things you crave at the moment.

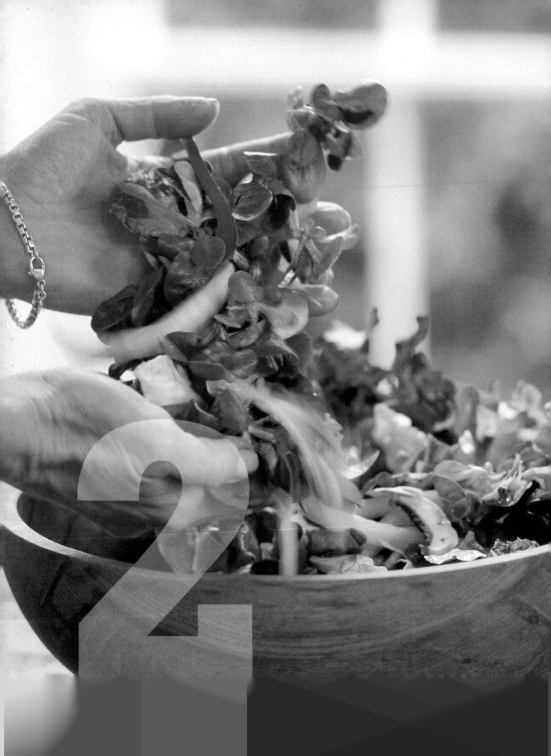

What
you eat...

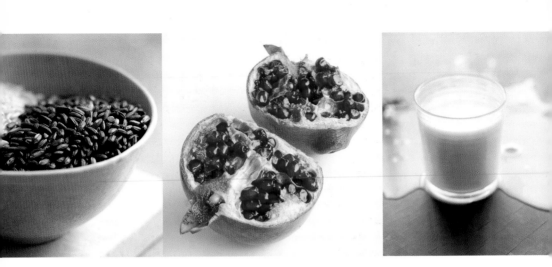

A balanced diet

Dietary advice has become a minefield – food scares, clever marketing campaigns and complicated food labels often create confusion rather than clarity. It makes sense to eat a balanced diet, but what exactly is that? A balanced diet for someone trying to lose weight will be different from that of a serious marathon runner. No single food delivers all the nutrients the body requires to stay healthy, and a good diet should include a variety of foods from all the major food groups.

Foods contain five classes of nutrients: carbohydrates, fats, proteins, vitamins and minerals. They also contain water, which is essential for all your body's processes, and fibre, which is necessary to keep your digestive system functioning smoothly. Carbohydrates, fats and proteins provide the substratum the body needs to give it energy. These are called macronutrients. Vitamins and minerals have no calorific value, but are nevertheless essential for the breakdown of macronutrients.

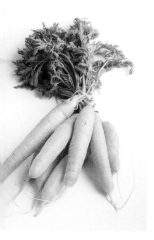

CARBOHYDRATES

What they are?

Carbohydrates form the backbone of our diet. Fruit, vegetables, simple sugars such as biscuits and cakes, and starchy carbs such as potatoes, rice and bread are all carbohydrate-rich foods. Carbohydrates are usually classified as either simple or complex, according to their chemical structure. Recently, carbohydrates have been classified according to the Glycaemic Index as well (see page 22).

Why you need them?

Carbohydrate-rich foods supply the body with its primary source of fuel – glucose. Glucose is a type of sugar that the body can easily use and transport (when we talk about blood sugars, we are actually talking about our blood glucose levels). Glucose can also be stored in the muscles as glycogen and is the main source of fuel for the nervous system and brain. Carbohydrates must be present for us to burn body fat; but any excess calories from carbohydrates will be converted to and stored as body fat in our fat cells.

How much do we need?

Some health institutions and nutritionists recommend that we obtain between 50 and 65 per cent of our calorie intake from carbs, but more recent guidelines are based on body weight per kilogram: 4–5g of carbohydrate per kg of body weight for healthy, active people. The recent popularity of high-protein, low-carb diets has misled many of us into cutting out carbs altogether. A moderate reduction is probably beneficial to weight loss, but banning carbs totally is ultimately detrimental to health and energy levels. Implementing a 'Carb Curfew', however – avoiding starchy carbs after 5pm – can be an effective, simple and easy way to achieve a better balance of nutrients

INTRODUCE THE CARB CURFEW

Carb Curfew means no starchy carbs – bread, pasta, rice, potatoes or cereal – after 5pm. Don't panic – you can incorporate a whole variety of nutritious foods in your evening meal, including lean meat and fish, fruit, vegetables, pulses and dairy products, and come up with something absolutely delicious! (see page 43)

WHAT IS THE GLYCAEMIC INDEX?

The Glycaemic Index (GI) ranks carbohydrate-containing foods according to their effect on the body's blood-glucose levels, and is therefore an extremely useful tool in our daily quest to keep energy levels balanced. Eating high-GI foods causes a 'sugar spike' as the body thinks we have eaten a large quantity of food and responds by releasing a large quantity of insulin into the bloodstream, which in turn disperses the food-glucose and a lot more, resulting in a dip in our blood glucose levels and hunger pangs all over again!

Low-GI foods have a value of less than 55, moderate-GI foods between 56 and 69, and high-GI foods have GI more than 70. The ratings are based on ingestion of 50g.

SOME GI COMPARISONS

Breads		Carb Foods	
Baguette	95	White rice	87
Gluten-free bread	90	Baked potatoes	85
Black rye bread	76	Chips	75
Bagels	72	Taco shells	68
White rolls	61	Polenta	68
Granary bread	61	Couscous	65
Stoneground bread	59	Basmati rice	58
Sourdough bread	57	Egg noodles	46
Pitta bread	57	Durum-wheat spaghetti	41
Oatcakes	54	Mung bean noodles	39
Rye bread	51	Pearl barley	25
Pumpernickel	50		
Fruit tea bread	47		

Desserts		Drinks	
Rice pudding	81	Glucose drink	95
Sponge cake with cream	67	Beer	88
Vanilla ice cream	61	Fizzy orange drink	68
Banana	55	Lemon squash	66
Plain yoghurt	46	Cola	53
Orange	44	Orange juice	50
Custard	43	Apple juice	40
Apple	38	Tomato juice	38
Fruit yoghurt	33	Skimmed milk	32
Cherries	22	Tea	0
		Water	0

FATS

What they are?

The fat in our food is the most concentrated source of energy, providing 9 calories per gram, more than twice as many as either protein or carbohydrate. Foods such as butter, oils, nuts, cheese and coconuts are all rich sources of fat. There are three main sub-groups, divided according to their chemical structure: saturated, polyunsaturated and monounsaturated.

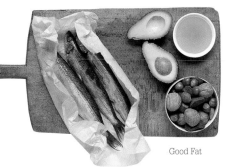

Good Fat

Why we need them?

It is important to stress that some fat is crucial for good health. Certain foods supply the fat-soluble vitamins A, D, E and K, as well as some essential fats, which the body cannot make for itself. Fat helps us to transport important antioxidants and to produce key hormones that regulate various body processes. If we cut out all fat in our diet, we would be depriving ourselves of vital nutrients.

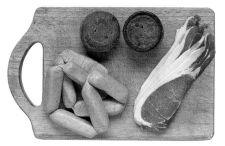

Bad Fat

SATURATED FATS

These are the least healthy, and have no useful function. Eating too much saturated fat is associated with an increased risk of heart disease. When we eat food that is high in saturated fat, the simplest thing for our body to do with it is transport it to the fat cells, and dump it there. Quite simply, the fat cells welcome the saturated fat we eat with open arms – they get bigger and bigger, our clothes get tighter and tighter and our health risks get higher and higher. Saturated fats include butter, lard, cheese and fat on meat.

POLYUNSATURATED FATS

These essential fats help us to burn energy from other foods such as proteins and carbohydrates. They play an important role in the healthy functioning of our body before what remains of them is transported to the fat cells and stored. They are subdivided into two groups:

Omega 3 essential fats: These are found in oily fish such as salmon, herring, sardines, trout, pilchards and mackerel, flaxseed and pumpkin seed. They are thought to help to prevent atherosclerosis, lower blood pressure and reduce blood fat (making the blood less sticky and thereby less susceptible to clotting). Eating three servings of oily fish a week, or using flaxseed oil in your salad dressing will help you hit your Omega 3 fatty acid quota.

Omega 6 essential fats: These are found mainly in hemp, pumpkin, sunflower, safflower, sesame and corn oil. About half of the oils found in these seeds come from Omega 6 fatty acids. They help prevent blood clots, lower blood pressure, maintain water balance in the body and stabilise blood sugar levels. However, excessive consumption may reduce beneficial high-density lipoproteins or HDLs, and exacerbate the damage done by potentially cancer-causing free radicals.

MONOUNSATURATED FATS

These are regarded as the most healthy fats, partly because research has shown that Mediterranean diets, rich in olive oil, are associated with the lowest risks of heart disease. However, bear in mind that a tablespoon of olive oil has the same number of calories as a tablespoon of melted lard!

STORAGE AND COOKING

- Keep flaxseed oil in a cupboard, as it can be damaged by exposure to light.
- Omega 3 fats can be damaged by excessive heat, so avoid cooking with these fats at high temperatures.

Monounsaturated fats are liquid at room temperature and because they are more stable than polyunsaturated fats, are a better choice for cooking oil. Rapeseed oil also contains monounsaturated fat.

TRANS/HYDROGENATED FATS

You may well have come across the term 'trans fats' or 'hydrogenated fats'. These fats are particularly unhealthy. They often started out as polyunsaturated fat, but after processing at very high temperatures, their chemical structure made them less stable and they became damaged. Consumption is associated with an increased risk of cancers and heart disease. They are found in margarine and processed foods so beware of the word 'hydrogenated' on food labels.

Type of fat	Where you find it	Health Rating
Monounsaturated fats	Olive oil, Canola, Olives, Nuts, Avocados	Excellent
Polyunsaturated	Corn oil, Sunflower oil, Sesame oil, Seeds	Good
Saturated fats	Butter/dairy products, Lard, Meat	Unhealthy: restrict to
	Eggs, Hydrogenated fats,	less than 10g a day
Hydrogenated fats	Vegetable shortening, Palm oil, Margarine	Bad: avoid these

According to new dietary recommendations, fat should constitute no more than 30 per cent of total calorie intake, and 10 per cent or less should come from saturated sources. If you are adhering to a 1,600-calorie a day diet, for example, this equates to 50–60g of fat per day in total, of which a maximum of 20g should be saturated.

PROTEINS

What they are?

Proteins are made up of chains of amino acids. There are hundreds of amino acids in nature, but only 23 are important to humans, and of these, 8 are termed 'essential', as we cannot manufacture them in the body, and therefore need to absorb them from the foods we eat. Meat, fish, pulses and dairy products are all foods with a high protein content.

Why you need them?

Proteins are essential for tissue repair, maintenance and growth, making up part of every cell in the body. A regular supply of protein is required for growth processes, and to repair bodily wear and tear. Protein can be divided into two groups: dairy products, which include milk, cheese and yoghurt, and non-dairy sources, which include meat, fish, nuts, seeds and eggs, pulses and beans. The important role that protein plays means that it is much harder for the body to store excess protein as fat.

How much do we need?

The Foods Standards Agency recommends that we obtain 15 per cent of our energy from protein. This amount is adequate for health purposes, but a higher intake is preferable if you want to restrict your calorie intake. Another way of determining your protein needs is by body weight: guidelines suggest aiming for 0.75g of protein per kg of body weight, so if you weigh 70kg you eat 52.5g of protein a day. It is important, however, that this is obtained from fish, lean meat sources, nuts and seeds, and balanced with plenty or fruits and vegetables.

Protein in the vegetarian diet

If you are a vegetarian or vegan, you will need to take a little more care with your protein intake, as plant protein sources (such as legumes, nuts and seeds) may not contain all the amino acids you need. It is therefore important to ensure that you get a good mix of different kinds of plant proteins.

Protein for athletes

If you are an athlete or involved in regular intense exercise, you will have a greater protein requirement, as extra protein is needed for muscle repair and recovery after training. However, studies have shown that you only need between 1.2–1.4g per kg of body weight to meet the demands of an average strength or endurance training programme: any amount above this provides no additional benefit.

DIETARY FIBRE

What it is?

Dietary fibre is the indigestible part of our food that helps our digestive system to function smoothly. There are two types of dietary fibre: soluble and insoluble.

SOLUBLE FIBRE

Dissolved in water, this forms a gel. Found in fruits, vegetables, legumes and oat bran, it helps reduce cholesterol when consumed as part of a diet low in saturated fat. Soluble fibre can also help control blood sugar levels.

INSOLUBLE FIBRE

This fibre cannot dissolve in water, but instead absorbs water as it passes through the body and contributes to faecal bulk. It's found in fruits, vegetables, whole grains and wheat bran.

Why we need it?

A high-fibre diet is important for several reasons: it can give your energy levels a boost, and helps lower the risk of diabetes, heart disease and possibly cancer. And – probably most important to you right now – it can help you to control your weight. Fibre slows digestion and makes you feel full, so it's a useful tool to use – but it will take a minimum of six servings of fruits and veggies and three servings of whole grains daily to meet recommendations.

Studies show that certain types of fibre lower cholesterol, normalise blood sugar in diabetics and, of course, help with digestive regularity. Regular

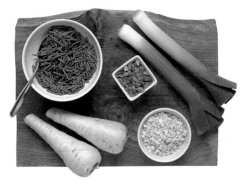

movements are not only important for bowel health but also improve mood.

HEALTHY EATING AND WEIGHT MANAGEMENT

Getting your head around nutrients need not be confusing: the most important thing is to ensure calorie intake is managed while you're still consuming proper levels of essential nutrients. Select a variety of foods, especially those that are nutrient-dense yet low in calories.

And remember:
- Eat lots of fruits and vegetables
- Fill up on fibre
- Avoid saturated fats
- Drink lots of water
- Choose lean proteins

VITAMINS AND MINERALS

Vitamins and minerals are vital components in our daily diet. While they provide no direct energy in the form of calories, they do play a very important role, as they are essential in the breakdown of macronutrients for the release of energy.

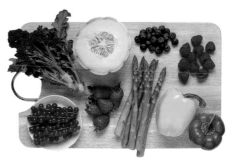

Since they only need to be consumed in small quantities, they are often referred to as 'micronutrients'. To help ensure that you are getting an adequate supply of vitamins and minerals, have a look at the quick-reference table on pages 30–31, which will inform you of the benefits of your favourite fruits, vegetables and other foods. Remember: food doesn't just meet your energy needs, but can directly affect your health and looks as well. Some diets advise you to take vitamin/mineral supplements while you are following them, but I always find this suspicious. A good balanced diet with fresh, unprocessed foods should provide the micronutrients you need, unless you are recovering from illness, pregnant or elderly.

JUICING

Juicing fruits and vegetables is a great way to get an antioxidant blast as well as helping you to fulfil your fruit and vegetable quota. While your palate will eventually grow to savour all-veggie juices, they can be tough for beginners. These easy-to-love recipes add fruit for natural sweetness.

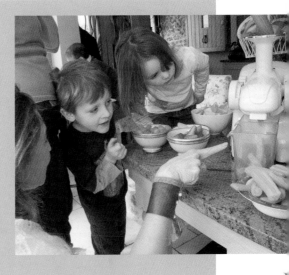

The Basic Cocktail: juice 3 carrots, 2 stalks celery, a 2.5cm piece of ginger and half an apple. It's a good souce of betacarotene and zinc, and boosts the immune system.

The Pick-me-up: juice 3 carrots, 2 fennel stalks with leaves and half a lemon. Relieves fatigue and releases feel-good brain chemicals.

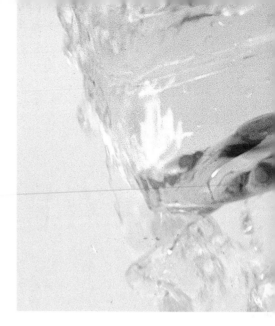

WATER

No natural resource is undervalued as much as fresh water. Nothing will have a greater immediate impact on your energy levels. If you drink less than eight glasses (2 litres) of water a day, your body may be chronically dehydrated. You will lack energy and your brain will misinterpret this tiredness and crave a sugary energy boost. Don't think you can quench your thirst with tea, coffee or colas – these will leave you dehydrated as well. Pure, clean water is the best drink of all.

Why is water important?

Water is crucial to every single process that occurs in our bodies. Every cell is bathed in water and every chemical or physiological reaction in our body requires its presence. If your body is even slightly dehydrated, you are asking it to perform in an environment that is not totally supportive to what it needs to do.

Why is water particularly important for weight management?

Water swells food cells and helps our body take up vital nutrients. It also makes us feel more satisfied. It bulks up food, stretching the stomach wall and sending messages to the brain telling us we are full. In addition, the water content in blood helps the absorption and transportation of all the nutrients, vitamins and minerals we have consumed (fat can only be broken down in the presence of water), and flushes waste products away. This is essential for your weight loss journey, because when you make the change to healthier eating, your body will initially produce more toxins, which will need to be flushed out.

Water also retrains your thoughts from hunger to thirst. The hypothalmus, the regulatory part of the brain, sends out messages telling us whether we are hungry or thirsty; sadly, however, if we become dehydrated, we lose the ability to understand the true message our hypothalamus is sending us.

How much should I drink?

Research suggests we need 1ml of fluid per calorie we consume. So if your average daily intake is 1,600 calories, you need a minimum of 1.6 litres of water. While a healthy diet containing lots of fruit and vegetables can provide a proportion of this fluid, we should supplement these sources with drinking water itself.

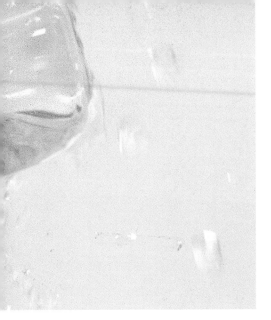

Why we need it?

We do need a certain amount of salt for our bodies to function smoothly – to keep nerve pathways working and to maintain our muscles. But too much salt has been clearly linked with hypertension (it raises blood pressure), which in turn increases the risk of heart disease or stroke (Britain's biggest killers). It is currently thought that we are each consuming in the region of 9g of salt a day, which is about 2 teaspoons. The Food Standards Agency is so alarmed by this figure that it is lobbying the food industry to reduce the amount of salt in processed food.

How much do we need?

Everyone should lower their sodium intake to 1,500mg daily (half a teaspoon of salt contains about 1,200mg of sodium). Try cooking with spices, herbs, lemon and salt-free seasoning blends to reduce sodium intake – and remember to read those labels.

And when?

Spread your water intake evenly throughout the day. If you're observing the 2-litre recommendation, that's a half-litre by lunchtime, a further litre by late afternoon and the remainder in the evening. You may find that initially this new regime will have you running to the loo, but as your body adjusts, the effect will wear off.

SODIUM AND SALT

From a health perspective, the amount of salt in our food is something we should all be aware of.

What it is?

Sodium is a calorie-free mineral that works its way into the diet in the form of salt. But we are not just talking saltshaker here – it is estimated that about 75 per cent of the sodium in our diet comes from processed foods.

CHOOSE SEA SALT

While table salt (sodium chloride) is responsible for raising blood pressure and causing heart problems, natural sea salt is health-promoting, since it contains many other minerals, including magnesium and calcium. It is the healthy alternative to sodium chloride, so use it when cooking and on food instead of table salt. Up to 5g (a teaspoon) per day is considered safe.

Vitamin	Found in	Functions in the body
Vitamin A (retinol)	Dairy products, green leafy vegetables, yellow and orange fruits, fortified cereals and oatmeals	Promotes healthy growth, maintains vision, skin cells, gut and respiratory tract.
Vitamin B1 (thiamin)	All vegetables, fortified cereals and oatmeal, whole grains, rice and pasta, meat	Maintenance of healthy nervous system, heart and growth. Involved in carbohydrate metabolism and energy production.
Vitamin B2 (riboflavin)	Green leafy vegetables, whole grains, organ meats	Helps the body release energy from protein, fats and carbohydrates during metabolism.
Vitamin B3 (niacin)	Fortified cereals and oatmeal, meat and poultry	Involved in carbohydrate, protein and fat metabolism.
Vitamin B6 (pyridoxine)	Whole grains, meats, poultry, fish	Aids both glucose and protein metabolism and energy production, maintains healthy nervous system. Important in resistance to infection.
Vitamin B12 (cobalamin)	Meat, seafood	Aids cell development, functioning of the nervous system and the metabolism of protein and fat.
Vitamin C (ascorbic acid)	Citrus fruits, berries	Essential for structure of bones, cartilage, muscle and blood vessels, helps maintain capillaries and gums and aids iron absorption.
Vitamin D (calciferol)	Dairy products, fish	Aids bone and tooth formation, helps maintain healthy functioning of the heart and nervous system.
Vitamin E (alpha-tocopherol)	Green leafy vegetables, fortified cereals and oatmeal, grain products, vegetable oils, nuts	Protects blood cells, body tissue and essential fatty acids from damage or destruction in the body.
Vitamin K	Green leafy vegetables, fruits, grain products, vegetable oils, nuts	Protects blood cells, body tissue and essential fatty acids from damage or destruction in the body.
Biotin	Fortified cereals and oatmeals, grain products, vegetable oils, nuts, whole grains, organ meats	Essential for blood clotting.

Vitamin	Found in	Functions in the body
Calcium	Milk and milk products	Essential for healthy bones and teeth. Important in muscle contraction and the transmission of nerve impulses.
Chromium	Whole grains, corn oil, clams, brewer's yeast	Important in glucose metabolism (energy), increases effectiveness of insulin.
Folate (folacin, folic acid)	Green leafy vegetables, organ meats	Aids genetic material development, involved in red blood cell production, and strengthens immune system
Iodine	Legumes, nuts, oysters, organ meats, seafood	Formation of red blood cells, bone growth and health. Works with Vitamin C to form elastin. Component of hormone thyroxine which controls metabolism.
Iron	Legumes, meats	Essential in red blood cell formation. Improves blood quality, increases resistance to stress and disease.
Magnesium	Green vegetables	Acid/alkaline balance, important in metabolism of carbohydrates, minerals and sugar.
Manganese	Whole grains, nuts	Enzyme activation, carbohydrates and fat production, sex hormone production, skeletal development.
Pantothenic acid	All vegetables, fruits, whole grains, meats	Aids the release of energy from fats and carbohydrates.
Phosphorus	Milk and milk products, eggs, grains, meat, poultry, fish	Important role in the delivery of energy to all cells, and formation of bones and teeth.
Potassium	All vegetables (particularly potatoes and tomatoes), lean meats	Maintenance of body fluids, controls activity of heart muscle, nervous system and kidneys.
Selenium	Grains, seafood, organ meats, lean meats	Protects body tissues against oxidative damage from radiation, pollution and normal metabolic processing.
Zinc	Eggs, whole grains, seafood, organ meats, lean meats	Involved in digestion and metabolism, important in development of reproductive system, aids healing.

YOUR HEALTHY EATING SHOPPING LIST – THE BASICS

It's a good idea to make several copies of this list. Mark items as you run out of them and add non-essentials under 'Miscellaneous'.

Shopping List

Fruit and vegetables
Apples
Aubergine
Bananas
Broccoli
Cabbage (green or red)
Carrots
Cauliflower
Celery
Courgettes
Cucumbers
Fresh greens
Garlic
Grapefruit
Grapes
Lemons
Melons
Mushrooms
Onions
Oranges
Parsley
Peppers
Plums
Squash
Sweet potatoes

Meat and fish
Bacon (pork or turkey) and ham (lean)
Beef (lean minced, various lean steaks)
Chicken (skinless breasts and
    bone-in parts)
Lamb (chops and minced)
Pork (chops)
Salmon fillets
Haddock or other white fish fillets
Prawns
Turkey (breast, minced)

Shopping List cont'd

Baking aisle
Brown sugar or brown sugar substitute
Cocoa powder (unsweetened)
Olive oil
Sesame oil
Coconut (unsweetened)
Dried fruits (apricots, raisins)
Nuts (almonds, macadmia, pecans,
    pine nuts, pistachios, walnuts)
Peanuts, unsalted, dry-roasted
Sea salt and black pepper
Dried herbs and spices
Seeds (sesame, sunflower, pumpkin)

Canned and jarred foods
Reduced-salt stock
Dried or canned beans (black, brown
    lentils, chickpeas, pinto, red kidney,
    white)
Fish (anchovies, salmon, sardines, trout
    fillets, tuna in spring water or light
    olive oil, pilchards, skips, crab)
Fruit in fruit juice (no sugar added)
Mild green chilli peppers
Tinned tomato products
Olives
Roasted red peppers

Condiments and sauces
All-fruit spread
Hot-pepper sauce
Marinara sauce (low-sugar)
Mayonnaise (no added sugar,
    reduced fat)
Various mustards
Dried chilli flakes
Nut butter, natural
Pesto

Shopping List cont'd

Soy sauce (reduced salt)
Vinegar (cider, balsamic, red/white wine)
Thai sweet chilli sauce
Mirin (Japanese rice wine vinegar)

Rice, pasta, grains
Brown rice
Porridge oats
Pinhead oats
Pearl barley
Quinoa
Wholewheat couscous
Wholewheat pasta

Frozen foods
Broccoli
Corn
Fruit (no sugar added)
Green beans
Peas
Spinach

Bread products
Tortillas (corn, wholewheat)
Wholegrain crispbreads
Wholemeal bread

Refrigerated foods
Butter (preferably light)
Cheese (Cheddar, Parmesan, reduced fat
    cream cheese, cottage)
Eggs
Reduced-fat margarine (avoid
    trans/hydrogenated fats)
Milk, skimmed or semi-skimmed
Orange juice
Yoghurt (low-fat bio, plain)

WHEN SHOPPING, ALWAYS READ THE LABEL!

Food labels can be very misleading, both in terms of establishing exactly how many calories you are consuming and in the terminology they use. For example, peanut butter labels may read 'cholesterol free' – but peanut butter never had any cholesterol in the first place! And 'cholesterol free' does not mean 'fat free'. Some labels will boast 'No Added Fat' on their 'healthy' cereal box, although in fact the contents may well have been processed with coconut or palm oil, both high in saturated fat.

Here are some things to look out for:

- Look at total fat intake and not just saturated fat. Any fat, healthy or not, provides 9 calories per gram.
- Just because it says 'low fat' on the front does not necessarily mean it is a low-fat food. An apple is a naturally low-fat food while 'low-fat' mayo is not!
- Avoid trans fats by looking for the term 'hydrogenated'. The higher up the list you see this term, the more unhealthy fats there are in the food.
- It may say 'reduced fat' on the label but do check out the total calories – the extra flavour may come by way of added sugars and processed flavourings.
- Consider buying a ready-reference calorie counter or using one on-line.

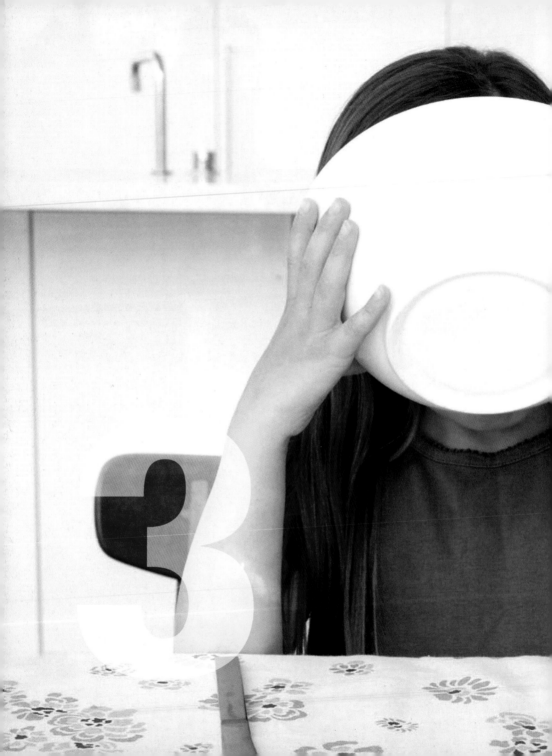

How you eat

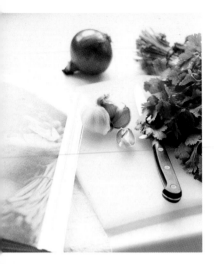

How to cut calories... in 7 easy steps

The following principles will help you reach your weight loss destination. Remember that people who've got there and stayed there do not continually count calories, but they are calorie aware – and you will start to develop these skills too as you put the principles in practice.

1. INTRODUCE THE CARB CURFEW

Carb Curfew means no starchy carbs – bread, pasta, rice, potatoes or cereal – after 5pm. Don't panic – you won't feel as if you're about to starve, since there are still plenty of filling foods to eat. You can incorporate a whole variety of nutritious foods in your evening meal, including lean meat and fish, fruit, vegetables, pulses and dairy products, and come up with something absolutely delicious! Turn to the dinner recipe ideas on pages 74–95 and you'll see what I mean.

　　Many of my clients consider the Carb Curfew to be the single most important tool in their weight management success and I know it can help you too. The Carb Curfew helps you control your insulin levels, which means it's easier to stabilise your energy levels – important for weight loss.

Why?

■ It's an easy way to create an Energy Gap! You will be cutting down on calories and filling up slow-releasing, energy-providing pulses, so you'll feel less hungry and more energetic.

■ Substituting fruit and vegetables instead of rice or pasta will increase your vitamin and mineral intake, which is important for the breakdown of macronutrients.

■ It reduces bloating. As your body digests and stores carbohydrate, it breaks it down into glucose and either stores it as glycogen in the muscles or as fat in the fat cells. Storing those starchy carbs as glycogen is your body's preferred choice but to do this it has to store three units of water with every one unit of glycogen. The net result is a bloated tummy.

- It prevents food hangovers. If you stuff your face at night, you will wake up with a 'food hangover' and won't want breakfast. By the evening, you'll be starving again.

2. STOP PORTION DISTORTION

One of the main reasons we are gaining weight is that we are over-eating. Portion sizes in restaurants and fast-food outlets have increased eightfold in the past 20 years, as companies vie with each other to lure consumers with ever-bigger promises of value for money. When serving sizes are bigger and bigger, it becomes difficult to decide what a 'normal' portion is.

Why?
- It allows you to eat the things you like, as long as you control the amount you're eating.
- Excess food means excess calories.

3. INCLUDE PROTEIN IN EVERY MEAL

Although many nutritionists are still wary about the potential dangers of high-protein diets, consuming slightly more protein than you normally would can be an effective tool for weight loss, as it helps you feel fuller for longer.

Why?
- Protein contains an essential amino acid called leucine, a muscle regulator vital to weight loss that can be obtained only from protein sources.

STOPPING PORTION DISTORTION – A FEW TIPS

Weighing out the correct portion of food can be a bore, so let's make things simple. To keep your meals in check, compile a handy Portion Distortion basket in your kitchen. Put in it some everyday items that are the same size as the portion of food you should be eating. Soon you'll become familiar with the sizes, so you'll be able to stop Portion Distortion wherever you are – in a restaurant you can order what you want but only eat as much as the size of the healthy portion. Watching the size of your portions is an invaluable piece of weight-loss advice. Use the following objects to judge the portion size you should be aiming at.

Think...	For...
Two dice	Nuts and cheese
Deck of cards	Meat and fish
Teaspoon	Oils and fats
Tennis ball	Vegetables
Golf ball	Uncooked rice or coucous
Computer mouse	Cooked portion of starchy carbs

- Protein helps blunt the rise in blood sugar after a meal or snack, so it gives you staying power.
- Protein stimulates the release of dopamine, which is a brain transmitter that actually makes you feel more alert. It boosts concentration and curbs lethargy.

3. LOWER YOUR FAT INTAKE

There is continued debate over whether a low-fat diet (less than 25 per cent of total calories) contributes to successful weight loss because good sources of fat actually help your body burn off other calories. The important thing is to cut down on the bad fats but keep enough of the good ones.

Why?
- Research has found that simply lowering dietary fat intake promotes weight loss because you take in far fewer calories.
- High fat foods are not very filling, so you're more likely to over-eat, yet a small amount of fat provides a high number of calories. It's a lose–lose situation!

5. FRONT-LOAD YOUR DAY

Starve yourself all day in the belief that you are creating an energy gap, and you're heading for disaster: under-eating by day only leads to over-eating in the evening. Eat a good, slow-energy-releasing breakfast every day, however, and you'll be on the right track immediately. Don't worry – it doesn't have to be first thing in the morning.

Why?
- It helps stabilise your energy levels. When you are hungry you will find yourself unable to make sensible food choices, and when you start eating again you'll find it harder to tell when you've had enough.
- Eating your food when your body needs it will encourage you to spread your calories evenly throughout the day. This way, you'll burn more calories through the thermic effect of food, and you'll have lasting energy.

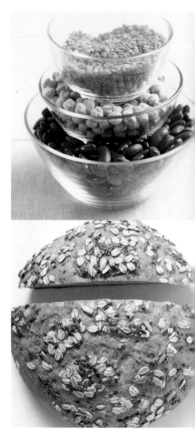

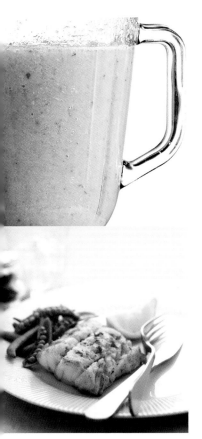

6. LIMIT ALCOHOL

Alcohol is a hidden pound-piler, although the good news is that losing weight doesn't mean giving up alcohol for life, just moderating your intake. From a health perspective, 'moderate' is equivalent to two drinks per day. From a weight perspective, if you can cut down on that, you will be making a significant saving in calories – and at particular stages of your weight loss journey cutting it out completely can be a big bonus.

Why?

- Alcohol is high in calories. A 500ml bottle of lager contains approximately 145 calories and a double measure of whisky (50ml) is 112 calories. Alcohol cannot be used directly by the muscles – it travels straight into the bloodstream, where it has to be metabolised before the body can convert it into fuel sources such as carbohydrate or fat. Research also suggests that a glass of wine may contribute more to your waistline than a slice of cake with the same calorie content.
- It weakens your calorie awareness, so self-discipline goes out the window and you tend to pick poor-quality foods.
- A study in the American Journal of Clinical Nutrition found that just a single glass of pre-lunch wine or beer left volunteers feeling less satisfied after their meal, and increased calorie intake over the next 24 hours.

7. HAVE MORE LIQUID-BASED FOODS

Try to incorporate more soups, juices and smoothies as well as water-based vegetables and fruit into your diet. Liquid-based food doesn't mean liquid lunches, however!

Why?

- Foods with a high water content help stave off hunger and make you feel full. Studies have shown that dieters who follow this advice tend to stick to their diet plan without feeling unsatisfied or deprived.

ALCOHOL AND YOUR HEALTH

The good news is that there are some health benefits to be had from drinking alcohol in moderate amounts. A recent study from the University of Alabama reported that moderate consumption of alcohol may decrease production and circulating levels by up to 20 per cent of a clotting protein called fibrinogen – high levels of which are associated with coronary artery, cerebrovascular and peripheral vascular diseases. Other research associates moderate alcohol intake with a lower risk of gallstones. Chronic heavy drinking, on the other hand, is a leading cause of several cardiovascular illnesses, including high blood pressure, as well as diseases of the liver and gastrointestinal organs. Research has also shown that it may be harmful to bones. A significant reduction in bone remodelling – the process of replacing old bone with new – occurs when alcohol is consumed in moderate or high amounts.

TIPS FOR HEALTHY DRINKING

- Watch the size of your glass! Most pubs and bars serve wine in 175ml or even 250ml glasses, but an official 'unit' of wine is actually just 125ml of 9 per cent alcohol wine. It's easy to go overboard without realising it if you drink from a larger glass, or if you drink stronger wine – a 125ml glass of wine with 12 per cent alcohol is actually 1.5 units. Half a pint of ordinary strength lager or bitter (3.5 per cent alcohol) and a single measure of spirits (40 per cent alcohol) are one unit each.
- The Department of Health guidelines stipulate that women should drink a maximum of 3 units per day and men 4 units, although their weekly guidelines are 14 units for women and 21 for men – so they assume that people will not drink their full quota every day.
- If you drink three units of red wine a day you are clocking up an extra 255 calories. If you drink four units of lager, you're consuming 400 calories. Three gin and diet tonics could mean an additional 255 calories a day – or 1,785 in a week. You'd have to do a lot of extra aerobic activity to burn all those off!
- While it's good to have a few alcohol-free days each week, don't 'save up' your units for a binge on Friday night – this overstresses the liver and is likely to lead to low energy levels and poor eating habits.
- Mix alcoholic drinks with soft drinks or water to prevent dehydration.
- Don't eat crisps or nuts – the salt will make you thirsty so you'll drink more.
- Do not drink on an empty stomach. This will slow down the rate at which your body can metabolise alcohol and you will feel drunk very quickly.
- If you are short, very overweight, run down or tired, your body will be less alcohol-tolerant. Women may also find their tolerance is lower while they are menstruating.

The Menu Plans

The Menu Plans have been devised so that you can choose from a selection of breakfasts, lunches, dinners and snacks grouped according to their calorie content (you'll find all the recipes in chapter 4). Make your choices from the lists so that in total they add up to your personal daily calorie limit.

Try to spread your calories evenly throughout the day. For example, if your new daily calorie intake is 1,800, you may choose to organise your calories in the following way:

- Breakfast = 500 calories
- Lunch = 500 calories
- Snack = 300 calories
- Dinner = 500 calories

REMEMBER TO EAT!

If you are not consuming enough calories, your metabolism will be alerted to the possibility of an imminent food shortage and possible starvation! It will automatically slow down as the self-preservation instinct kicks in (that is, it gets better at holding on to the fat you have stored up). It's probable as well that you won't be getting enough of the nutrients you need – your health will suffer and your energy levels flag.

MEAL GOALS

When you're planning a day's meals, bear the following meal goals in mind, and choose foods that will keep your energy levels high all day long.

BREAKFAST

To help you become alert after your mini-hibernation. Make sure you eat some protein and a small portion of carbohydrates to round out your meal.

LUNCH

Head off a slump and stay sharp. Focus on your meal, eat a lot of vegetables, a deck-of-cards size portion of protein and a small portion of carbs. Watch your fat intake – it makes you sluggish.

AFTERNOON SNACK

To keep your spirits lifted until dinner. If you are having a stressful day, go the carb route to calm your nerves. Think effective hydration to keep your brain in gear. If you are dragging, then have a cup of coffee. Using caffeine strategically like this can be a great help, although you should try to reduce your overall intake.

DINNER

To put tension behind you, but not go to bed stuffed. Remember the Carb Curfew. If you get home hungry, have some vegetable soup: it will stave off the pangs until dinner, give you a head-start serving of vegetables and hydrate you.

Breakfast

200 calories or less

Banana-chocolate smoothie
(see page 110)

Moosewood sesame citrus
delight (see page 54)

Poached egg, tomato,
mushrooms and wholemeal
toast (see page 54)

Medium slice melon and 100g
plain cottage cheese

100g natural low-fat bio yoghurt
and 70g strawberries

1 slice wholemeal toast and a
medium banana

300 calories or less

Banana-sour cherry bread
(see page 111)

Poached egg on Marmite toast
(see page 54)

Fruity English muffin
(see page 56)

Cereal with milk and fruit
(see page 56)

Raspberry smoothie
(see page 56)

Breakfast on the go
(see page 56)

Around 400 calories

Natural yoghurt with granola
and apple purée (see page 55)

Date and pumpkin seed brunch
loaf (see page 51)

Pinhead oatmeal porridge with
raisins (see page 50)

Blueberry-yoghurt slush with
granola (see page 55)

Banana muffins (see page 52)

Peanut butter toast and a piece
of fruit (see page 56)

Lunches

300 calories or less

Stuffed baked potatoes with
sun-dried tomatoes

Marinated tuna steak with
mushroom and parsley salad
(see page 68)

Teriyaki tofu with red peppers
and houmus roll-up
(see page 64)

Lentil salad with lardons
(see page 70)

Open sandwich (see page 72)

400 calories or less

Caesar salad with Cajun grilled
chicken (see page 65)

Spicy fruity coleslaw with ham
in pitta bread (see page 61)

Baked trout with flaked almonds
and watercress salad
(see page 69)

Tuna, mushroom, parsley and
lemon stuffed pitta
(see page 60)

Grilled herring on oatmeal
(see page 67)

Pitta Niçoise salad
(see page 72)

500 calories or less

Italian-style mackerel
(see page 62)

Easy tuna melt (see page 72)
with a tossed green salad

Avocado and chicken wrap
(see page 72) and a glass
of fresh fruit juice

Lunch on the run
(see page 72) with an iced tea

A dish from the 300 or less
lunches plus one from the
200 or less desserts

Dinners

300 calories or less

Easy fish and prawn curry
(see page 79)

Aromatic summer salmon
with purple grape and
chilli mango salsa
(see page 89)

Mexican vegetable soup
(see page 90)

Roasted autumn veg with
soy-marinated tofu
(see page 84)

Asian-flavoured chowder
(see page 87)

400 calories or less

Gammon steak with Puy lentils
and stir-fried greens
(see page 94)

Chicken fillet en papillote
(see page 80)

Tray-baked citrus chicken with
lentils and rocket
(see page 83)

Teriyaki chicken on red onion
and mushrooms (see page 86)

500 calories or less

Healthy chicken nuggets
with easy baked chips
(see page 108)

Thai green curry (see page 76)

Chickpea and almond crêpes
(see page 95)

Chilli chicken and white bean
burgers (see page 93)

A dish from the 300 or less
dinners plus one from the 200
or less desserts

Snacks & Desserts

300 calories or less

Apple and a matchbox-sized
piece of Edam or feta cheese

300ml glass skimmed milk

Rhubarb and strawberry jelly
(see page 99)

Baked bananas en papillote
(see page 100)

Peaches baked with mascarpone
(see page 102)

2 fresh figs, or a peach or a cup
of cherries

400 calories or less

200ml glass skimmed milk with
2 small cubes dark chocolate

Banana-chocolate smoothie
(see page 110)

2 crispbreads with Marmite

Orange, mango and passion fruit
(see page 98)

Cinnamon-poached fruit
(see page 101)

Muesli bar

500 calories or less

Slice of date and pumpkin-seed
loaf (see page 51)

Banana muffin (see page 52)
with matchbox piece of cheese

Handful of dried fruits
and nuts

2 crispbreads spread with half
an avocado and topped with
cottage cheese

Mango and banana smoothie
(see page 57)

A small piece of chocolate chip
banana snack cake
(see page 103)

Healthy eating for children

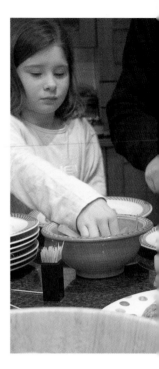

Exercise and activity are crucial to maintaining weight, and are an important part of a healthy lifestyle but it goes without saying that the food your children eat is equally important.

Children should be encouraged to enjoy healthy food, and to get pleasure from the experience of eating with friends and family. Good food keeps moods even, weight under control, helps them to learn and concentrate, encourages healthy growth and prevents disease. So healthy food should be a way of life, rather than a regime that is put into place every now and then. Remember: no child should ever be 'put on a diet'. It creates the wrong message and nurtures a template of failure.

JUNK FOOD

The temptation of junk food comes from all around them – not just from their friends but of course from advertising as well. But it's crucial that you combat it. Most importantly, remember that you are a crucial role model. If you relax with a packet of crisps, a chocolate bar and a glass of wine every evening, your kids will incite mutiny. Try to eat together, eat the same healthy foods, and keep the word 'diet' firmly away from your household.

We all like a treat from time to time, but you could help to redefine the word 'treat' if you're clever. Asparagus can be presented as a special dinner-time treat. A handful of ripe cherries and a little bowl to 'spit' the stones into is always popular. Multi-coloured vegetable crudités and their own little dish of dip will make many children happy.

Don't use the word 'treat' to define sweets or crisps. Instead, you could talk about 'sometimes' foods; explain that these are not everyday foods, because they're not very good for you, but that your child can have some from time to time so long as their diet is otherwise healthy. If you educate their tastebuds to enjoy fresh, natural tastes, they may even come to dislike the extremely salty or artificially sweet flavours of most types of junk food.

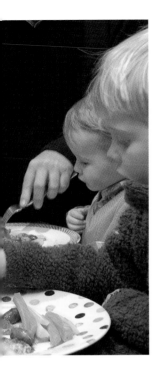

THESE TIPS ARE TRIED AND TESTED ON REAL FAMILIES – AND THEY WORK

- Make meal time family time. Keep to set times as much as possible. Eat at the table, turn off the television and talk about what you all did that day.
- Go hands-on! Get the kids involved in preparing nutritious meals. From babyhood, children are fascinated by the texture, colour and taste of food, and when they're old enough you can help them be creative with it. Healthy pizzas, kebabs, fruit sticks and salads are all easily undertaken, even by little ones.
- Make healthy choices easy choices. Always keep the fruit bowl visible and easy to reach. Fill the snack cupboard with muesli bars, low-fat biscuits or fruit snacks.
- Search the supermarket. Food companies are bringing out new healthy food for children every month. Check food labels (see page 33) and make a list of good options. As a guideline, go for foods with less than 10g of fat and 15g of sugar per 100g. Watch out too for salt and sodium.
- Make all food family food. While kids will undoubtedly squawk for the same food their peers are eating (the ubiquitous chicken nuggets or turkey twizzlers, for example), they'll also take great pride in eating what mum and dad eat. Every family member should eat the same meals, and be encouraged to try new dishes from time to time.
- Survey school food. Find out what food choices are available at your child's school. Do they have healthy options you can include on lunch orders? Is the school part of a healthy canteens programme? Can parents get involved to help increase the number of healthy options?
- Watch the fat talk. Avoid making negative comments about your child's weight. Even sometimes seemingly endearing terms can be damaging. Curb their 'fat talk' too.
- Don't choose unhealthy foods with a 'lower fat' or 'reduced sugar' content – they'll learn nothing about healthy eating if you serve the same junk with fewer unhealthy ingredients.
- Don't be tempted to go low-fat. Kids need fat to grow and develop. Simply serve a little less rather than low-fat brands.
- Offer small servings at first. They can always ask for more if they are hungry. Downsize the food portions the whole family eats.
- Provide milk or juice at the end of meal times, so they don't get full before they eat.

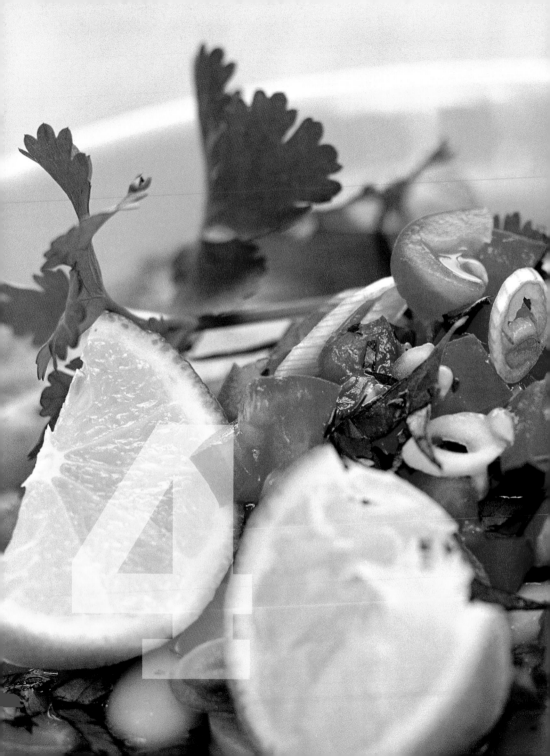

The recipes

There is a whole host of flavours, textures and taste sensations for you to enjoy. The nutritional information is given per serving for each dish. Always check how many people the recipe serves and divide the dish to get the correct portion size.

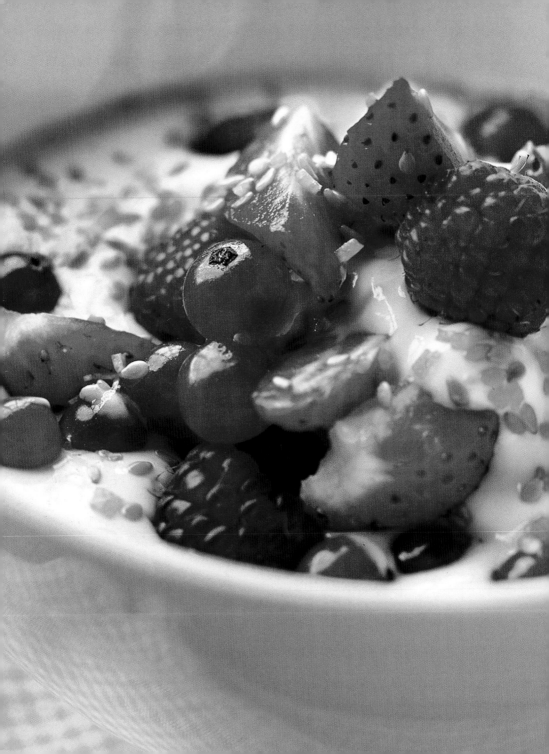

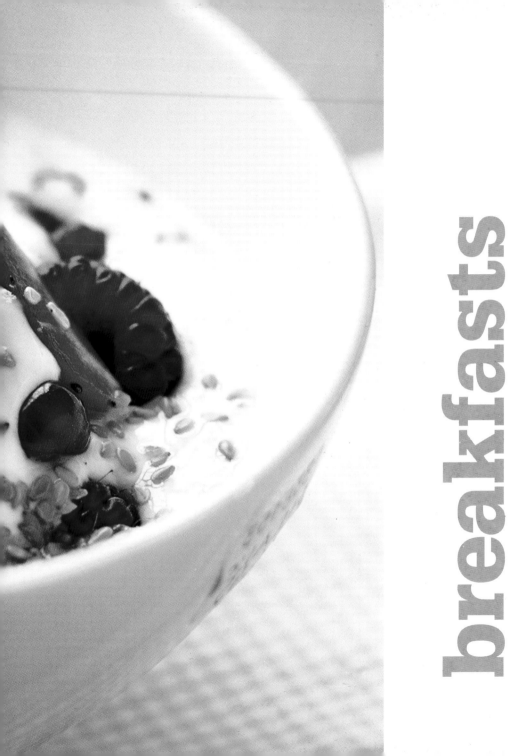

breakfasts

Pinhead oatmeal porridge with raisins

Oatmeal is full of slow-release carbohydrates to keep you going until lunchtime. If you can't find pinhead oatmeal, use regular rolled oats and don't worry about soaking them. The recipe below is designed to be easy to fit around your morning routine, and to save on washing up.

Serves 1 ▪ Prep time: 1 minute, plus 15 minutes soaking
Cooking time: 4–5 minutes

90g pinhead oatmeal
30g raisins
275ml boiling water

As you stumble blearily down to make a cup of tea, measure the oatmeal and raisins into a microwaveable bowl. When the kettle has boiled, pour the boiling water over the oatmeal-raisin mix and leave to soak. Go and get dressed.

When you're ready for breakfast, cover the bowl with clingfilm and microwave on high for 3 minutes. Stir, microwave for another 1½ minutes on high and then leave to stand for 3 minutes.

Serve with soya milk or semi-skimmed milk.

calories 414 ▪ fat 7.97 ▪ protein 13.21 ▪ carbohydrates 75.04

Date and pumpkin-seed loaf

This is delicious with a cup of herbal tea in the morning, with the dates and pumpkin seeds giving you fibre and lots of minerals to set you up for the day. It also freezes well, so slice it when it has cooled, layer the slices with baking parchment and wrap in a plastic bag so you can remove a single slice at a time.

Serves 8 ▪ Prep time: 15 minutes ▪ Cooking time: 25 minutes

200g fresh dates, stoned and roughly chopped
150g raisins
65g pumpkin seeds
225g self-raising flour
100g soft margarine
100g caster sugar
2 large eggs
125ml water (at room temperature)

Preheat the oven to 180°C/350°F/Gas Mark 4. Grease a 1lb loaf tin well. Put the dates and the raisins in a mixing bowl. In the saucepan, toast the pumpkin seeds over a medium heat (with no oil) until they begin to brown. Tip them over the dates and raisins. Sift the flour over this and mix well, to make sure that all the sticky bits of date are coated in flour.

Beat the margarine and sugar together, on a high speed, until the mixture is light and fluffy. Add the eggs and beat again. Add the flour/fruit mixture to the margarine/sugar mixture, pour the hot water over the top and mix with a wooden spoon until everything is incorporated.

Scrape into the prepared tin, level the top and bake for an hour. Check it after half an hour and put a layer of tin foil loosely over the top if it's browning too fast. A skewer inserted into the middle of the loaf should come out clean when it's ready. Remove it from the oven and leave it to cool down before tipping it out of the tin.

calories 422 ▪ fat 13.56 ▪ protein 6.5 ▪ carbohydrates 72.68

Banana muffins

A weekend treat when you feel like putting a little more time into preparing brunch. Two muffins, a little non-sugar fruit jam, a glass of prune juice and herbal tea makes a 400 kcal breakfast.

Serves 6 (makes 12 muffins) ▪ **Prep time: 15 minutes**
Cooking time: 25 minutes

200g unbleached white flour
½ tsp bicarbonate of soda
1 tsp baking powder
½ tsp ground cinnamon
½ tsp nutmeg
60g brown sugar
100g porridge oats
1 egg white
1 egg
2 tbsp sunflower oil
2 ripe bananas, mashed
50g low fat natural yoghurt
50g sultanas

Preheat the oven to 200°C/400°F/Gas Mark 6. Prepare a muffin tin with paper liners, cooking spray or a fine coat of oil.

Sift together the flour, bicarbonate, baking powder and spices and stir in the sugar. Process the oats in a blender and stir into the other dry ingredients. Beat the egg white for 3 minutes until increased in volume but not stiff. Stir in the egg, oil, bananas, yoghurt and sultanas. Fold the wet ingredients into the dry until just combined but not too homogeneous.

Spoon the batter into the muffin tin, and bake for 20–25 minutes until a skewer comes out clean (a length of spaghetti works just as well for testing). Allow to cool in the tin for 5 minutes, then turn out onto a cooling rack.

calories 337.33 ▪ fat 7.50 ▪ protein 10.12 ▪ carbohydrates 61.52

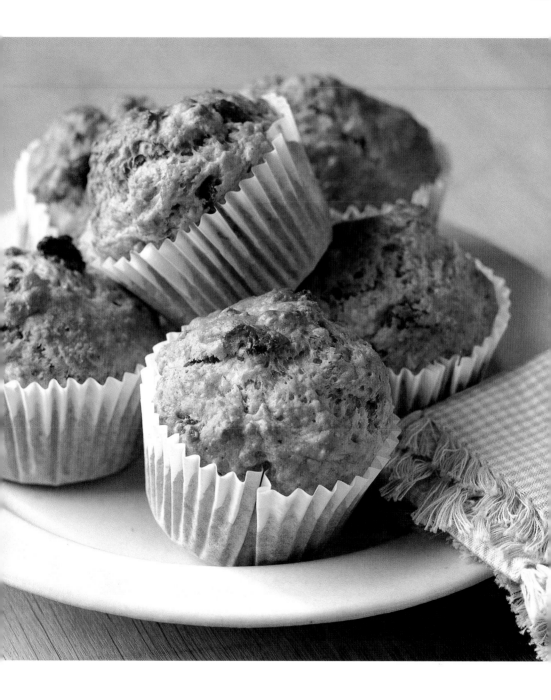

Moosewood sesame citrus delight

Moosewood is a famous American vegetarian restaurant, well known for its world food and innovative cooking. This is adapted from one of its recipes.

Serves 2 ▪ Prep time: 10 minutes ▪ Cooking time: 15 minutes

400g low-fat natural yoghurt
1 tbsp toasted sesame seeds
2 tbsp honey
1 tsp freshly grated orange peel
1 tsp freshly grated lemon peel
a pinch of salt
100g berries, e.g. strawberries or raspberries, to serve

Toast the sesame seeds on an un-oiled baking tray in a medium oven for 2–3 minutes. Cool, then combine all of the ingredients in a bowl, cover and chill for at least half an hour.

Serve topped with 100g of your favourite berries.

calories 116.75 ▪ fat 2.76 ▪ protein 5.85 ▪ carbohydrates 18.24

Poached egg on Marmite toast with orange juice

A classic. If you don't like Marmite or Vegemite then add a sprinkle of salt, and be generous with the pepper grinder.

Serves 1 ▪ Prep time: none ▪ Cooking time: 5 minutes

1 fresh hen's egg
1 slice brown bread
1 teaspoon Marmite or Vegemite (optional)
black pepper
200ml freshly squeezed orange juice

Simmer a little water in a small saucepan and toast the bread. Slide the egg into the simmering water and cook for about 2 minutes. Spread the Marmite, if using, on the toast. Remove the egg from the water, place it on the toast and season with pepper. Serve with a glass of freshly squeezed orange juice.

calories 227 ▪ fat 5.39 ▪ protein 8.94 ▪ carbohydrates 37.73

Natural yoghurt with granola and apple purée

Delicious, and so good for you. Serve with a cup of refreshing unsweetened herbal tea – lemon verbena is a good choice.

Serves 1 ▪ Prep time: 1 minute ▪ Cooking time: 5 minutes

1 medium eating apple, grated or sliced

100g low fat natural probiotic yoghurt

50g unsweetened muesli or granola

Stew the apple gently with a dessertspoon of water for 5 minutes until soft.

Sprinkle the yoghurt with the muesli or granola, and top with the stewed apple.

calories 378 ▪ fat 14.35 ▪ protein 12.86 ▪ carbohydrates 54.59

Blueberry-yoghurt slush with granola

If you can find fresh blueberries by all means use them, but the frozen ones work just as well – if not better – for this wonderfully purple breakfast.

Serves 1 ▪ Prep time: 1 minute ▪ Cooking time: none

100g low-fat natural probiotic yoghurt

100g fresh or frozen blueberries

50g muesli or granola

1 tbsp clear honey

Mix the yoghurt and blueberries together with a fork – how much you mix depends on how purple you like your food! Frozen blueberries will defrost as you mix them, but you might want to set the slush aside for a few minutes to warm up.

Place the slush in a serving bowl, top with the granola or muesli, and drizzle the honey over the top.

calories 412 ▪ fat 14.49 ▪ protein 13.08 ▪ carbohydrates 63.01

Quick Breakfasts all serve 1

Peanut butter toast

Two slices wholegrain seeded toast with 2 teaspoons peanut butter, a small sliced banana, and a 125ml glass of any natural fruit juice.

calories 349 ▪ **fat 10.65** ▪ **protein 10.24** ▪ **carbohydrates 58.65**

Fruity English muffin

Spread a toasted English muffin with 100g low-fat cream cheese and top with a sliced plum and a sprinkle of cinnamon.

calories 282 ▪ **fat 6.31** ▪ **protein 19.38** ▪ **carbohydrates 36.69**

Raspberry smoothie

Mix 1 teacup unsweetened soya or skimmed milk, 100g frozen or fresh raspberries (no added sugar), ½ banana, ½ cup silken tofu (you will find this at a health food shop in the chilled cabinet). Blend and go!

calories 236 ▪ **fat 7.79** ▪ **protein 14.06** ▪ **carbohydrates 31.85**

Breakfast on the go

Grab an apple (or fruit of your choice), 125g natural plain bio yoghurt and 20g nuts such as almonds or hazelnuts.

calories 258 ▪ **fat 12.45** ▪ **protein 11.01** ▪ **carbohydrates 28.92**

Cereal with milk

Bowl of 50g of your favourite wholewheat cereal sprinkled with a tablespoon wheatgerm, a teaspoon of crushed flaxseed and 50g blueberries, finished with ice-cold skimmed milk.

calories 260 ▪ **fat 1.79** ▪ **protein 12.79** ▪ **carbohydrates 57.92**

Or what about …

A large bowl of fresh fruit salad

with 100g natural low-fat bio yoghurt

215 calories

A large slice of melon

with 50g Bran Flakes, a slice of wholemeal toast with peanut butter
and 275ml skimmed milk

410 calories

A slice of orange

2 slices of toast with 1 tsp healthy margarine and honey,
and 25g Edam cheese

368 calories

200ml orange juice

50g Shreddies or other wholewheat cereal, a sliced banana, 1 slice toast,
1 tsp healthy margarine with 275ml skimmed milk

500 calories

1 poached egg and grilled tomato

50g poached mushrooms in 1 tbsp milk and a slice wholemeal toast
(165 calories).

25g porridge

soaked in 275ml skimmed milk, a grated apple and a handful of raisins
with a pinch of cinnamon

323 calories

A mango and banana smoothie

(1 banana, 1 mango, ½ pot natural low-fat bio yoghurt,
275ml skimmed milk and ice)

280 calories

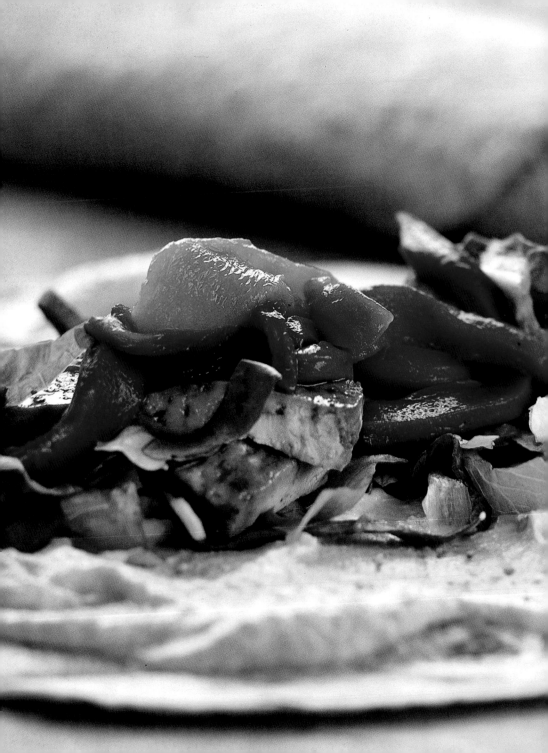

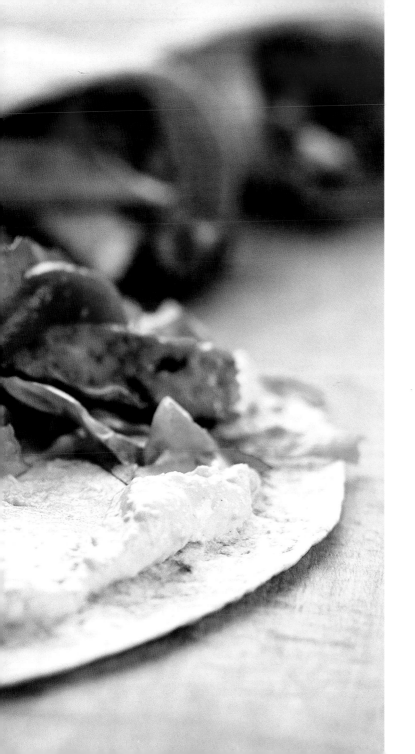

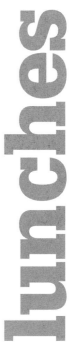
lunches

Tuna, mushroom, parsley and lemon stuffed pitta

This is the quick and easy 'cheat's version' of the more time-consuming Marinated tuna steak with mushrooms recipe on page 68.

Serves 2 ▪ **Prep time: 5 minutes** ▪ **Cooking time: none**

1 x 185g tin tuna in spring
water, drained

200g thinly sliced button
mushrooms

½ tbsp olive oil

100g flat-leaved parsley

juice of two lemons

salt and pepper

2 pitta bread

Flake the tuna into a bowl and break it up with a fork. Mix in the mushrooms, olive oil, parsley and lemon juice and add salt and pepper to taste.

Toast the pitta bread until it puffs up, then stuff it with the salad. Delicious.

calories 327.50 ▪ **fat 5.19** ▪ **protein 31.95** ▪ **carbohydrates 37.50**

Spicy fruity coleslaw
with ham, in pitta bread

Coleslaw can be both incredibly bland and far too vinegary, but here's a recipe to really make your tastebuds sit up. You can adjust the amounts of all the ingredients to suit your taste, but remember that it improves with time so don't make it too spicy or fruity to start with.

Serves 6 ▪ Prep time: 15 minutes ▪ Soaking time: at least 1 hour

125g dried apricots, roughly chopped

125g seedless sultanas

1 tsp brown sugar

1 tbsp white wine vinegar

125ml apple juice

125ml orange juice

1 tsp groundnut or sunflower oil

1 large head firm white cabbage

1 tsp salt

2.5cm fresh ginger, peeled and grated or finely chopped

1 small red onion, finely diced

½ red chilli (optional)

SERVE WITH

1 slice cooked ham per person

1 pitta bread per person

a few leaves of fresh coriander, chopped

Put the chopped apricots and sultanas into the mixing bowl and add the brown sugar. Pour over the vinegar, apple and orange juices and oil and stir well. Leave to soak for up to an hour, so the fruit plumps up and absorbs the other tastes. If you don't have the time, don't worry about it, but be prepared for slightly chewy fruit in the final dish.

Shred the cabbage as finely as you can and add it to the fruit along with the salt, ginger and red onion. If you're using the chilli then halve it lengthways and take the seeds out with a teaspoon before shredding it thinly and tossing it gently with the rest of the mixture. Leave the coleslaw in the fridge for as long as you can, for the flavours to develop.

When you want to eat, toast a pitta bread until it puffs up. Cut open the long end, lay a slice of ham inside, and fill with a portion of coleslaw. Sprinkle over the fresh coriander.

calories 333.33 ▪ fat 4.68 ▪ protein 16.30 ▪ carbohydrates 61.31

Italian-style mackerel

Unlike white fish, which store their 'good' oil in their livers, the oil of fish like mackerel, herrings and sardines is distributed throughout their bodies and makes them an ideal choice for healthy eating. Adding peas to the tomato sauce is an Italian classic and also gives you a portion of fibre- and vitamin-rich vegetables.

Serves 2 ▪ Prep time: 10 minutes ▪ Cooking time: 12 minutes

FOR THE FISH

2 medium mackerel fillets

olive oil spray

1–2 fresh lemons

FOR THE SAUCE

3 tsp olive oil

2 plump cloves garlic, peeled and finely chopped

60g black olives, pitted and finely chopped

1 tbsp parsley, finely chopped

3–4 anchovy fillets (50g), roughly chopped

1 glass red wine

230g tin chopped plum tomatoes

2 tbsp passata

lemon juice

sea salt and black pepper

150g frozen peas

3 tsp capers (optional)

good handful basil leaves, ripped

sea salt and freshly ground black pepper

To make the sauce, warm the olive oil in a medium-sized pan on a low heat. Gently cook the garlic, olives and parsley without browning. Add the anchovy fillets and stir in for about a minute. Turn the heat up to medium and add the wine; stir and let it simmer for about 2 minutes. Mix in the tomatoes and the passata, simmering and stirring for 4–5 minutes or longer on a low heat to intensify the flavours. Taste and season up as you go, with a good squeeze of lemon juice and black pepper.

While the sauce is cooking, pre-heat a griddle pan and lightly spray with olive oil. Rinse the mackerel fillet under a cold tap and pat dry with kitchen paper. Season the fish with a little sea salt and a good squeeze of lemon and spray the skin lightly with olive oil. Sear the fish on the hot griddle pan for about 45 seconds on each side. Turn the heat down to medium and cook for 3 minutes on each side. To check if it is cooked, gently slide the tip of a knife along the backbone to see if the flesh is opaque and firm.

Add the peas to the tomato sauce and then the capers, if using. Stir in half of the ripped basil leaves and spoon a generous pool of sauce onto 2 warmed plates. Perch the mackerel on top with a twist of lemon and the reserved basil leaves.

calories 464.5 ▪ fat 26.8 ▪ protein 28.3 ▪ carbohydrates 22.48

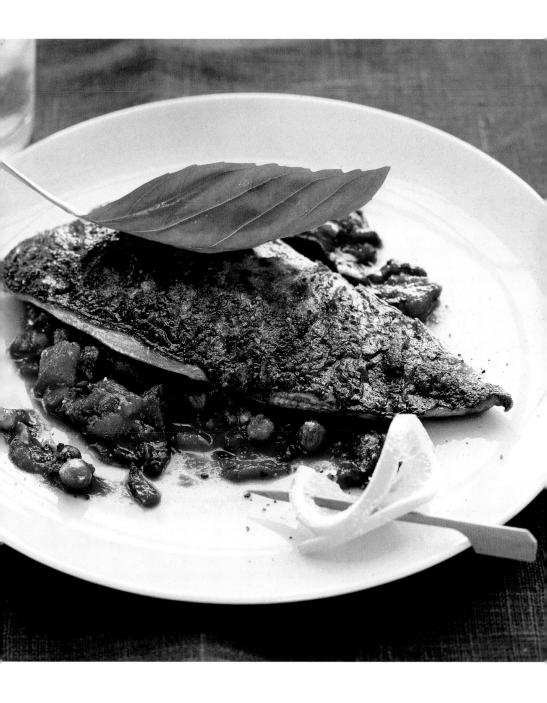

Teriyaki tofu with red peppers and houmous roll-up

Recipe illustrated on page 58

This is an ideal light lunch, and if you make the Teriyaki chicken (see page 86) the night before, you'll have plenty of sauce left over for this. Cover any leftover tofu in water and store it in the fridge: as long as you change the water every 24 hours it will keep for three days or so.

Serves 2 ▪ Prep time: 2 minutes ▪ Cooking time: 5 minutes

125g firm tofu

2 tbsp teriyaki sauce

50g roasted red pepper in a jar, well drained of its oil and thinly sliced

2 tbsp houmous

2 leaves fresh, cleaned and dried Boston or roundhead lettuce (or 2 leaves Romaine, shredded)

2 wholewheat tortillas

Cut the tofu into four generous centimetre-thick slices. Cover with teriyaki sauce, turning gently to ensure that all sides are coated. Turn the grill to high.

Place a sheet of tinfoil over your grillpan (tofu can fall apart when you move it). Lay the tofu slices at least 3cm apart from each other and then place under the grill. Leave them for 3 minutes then baste with any remaining marinade; turn them over, baste again and gril for another 2 minutes. It should take about 5 minutes in total, until they are soft.

While the tofu is grilling, place the tortillas in the oven beneath it, to catch the residual heat from the grill and soften them. When the tofu is cooked, take the tortillas out of the oven and spread the houmous thinly over them. Lay the lettuce on top of the houmous, put the red pepper and grilled tofu on top of that and roll up tightly.

calories 240.50 ▪ fat 7.94 ▪ protein 11.40 ▪ carbohydrates 37.84

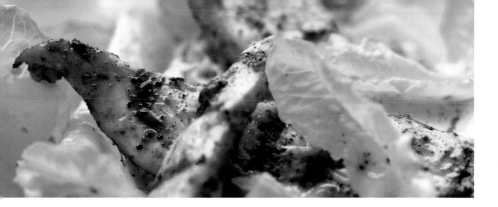

Caesar salad with Cajun grilled chicken

A non-traditional Caesar salad, but with a great flavour. There are several different brands of Caesar salad dressing available in the shops: taste it before serving, as you may like to jazz it up with a squeeze of lemon juice, half a teaspoon of mustard or half a teaspoon of soy sauce (or all three).

Serves 2 ▪ Prep time: 5 minutes ▪ Cooking time: 10 minutes

FOR THE CHICKEN

2 tbsp Cajun seasoning

1 tsp oil

2 x 100g skinless chicken breasts, cut into bite-sized chunks

FOR THE SALAD

15g freshly grated Parmesan cheese

4 tbsp Caesar salad dressing

1 tsp lemon juice (optional)

½ tsp mustard (optional)

½ tsp soy sauce (optional)

100g cos lettuce leaves torn into bite-size chunks

Mix the oil and Cajun seasoning together in a large bowl, then add the chicken and turn with a wooden spoon until all the pieces are well coated. Leave to marinate while you wash the lettuce and adjust the Caesar salad dressing to taste.

Put a ridged grill pan over a high heat. Add the chicken pieces and cook on both sides, pressing down with a spatula for a few seconds before turning them over and pressing down again. Leave to cool.

Toss the lettuce in the dressing and pile onto plates. Sprinkle the Parmesan on top and add the grilled chicken pieces with a twist of fresh black pepper.

calories 336 ▪ fat 19.75 ▪ protein 35.6 ▪ carbohydrates 2.8

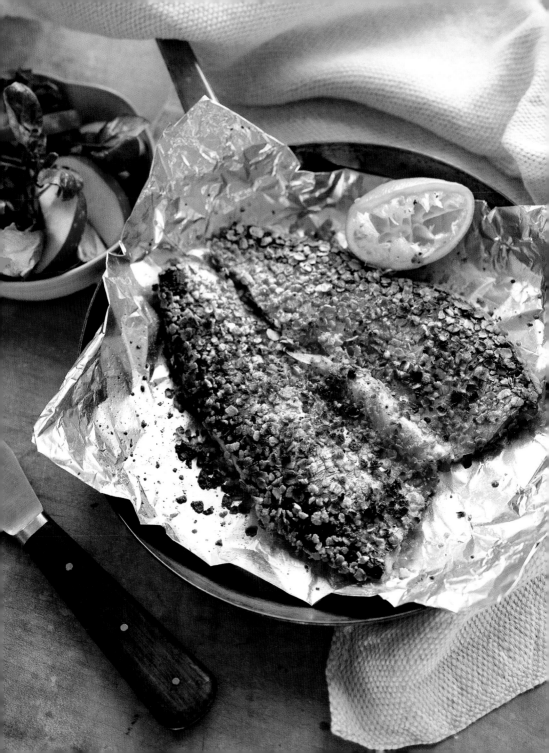

Grilled herring
on oatmeal

This is a healthy classic but so simple and delicious. Oatmeal is very high in fibre and iron and blends perfectly with the sweet, crunchy apple and peppery watercress salad.

Serves 2 ▪ Prep time: 2 minutes ▪ Cooking time: 10 minutes

2 herring, cleaned and butterflied (ask your fishmonger)
oatmeal coating
sea salt and black pepper
1 lemon

FOR THE SALAD
1 apple, sliced
100g (about 4 handfuls) watercress

Preheat the grill to medium and line the grill rack with a sheet of foil. Wipe or rinse the herring under cold water and pat dry with kitchen paper. Season the flesh with salt and pepper and sprinkle with lemon juice. Press the herring into a plate of oatmeal until well coated and grill flesh-side up for about 10 minutes, until golden.

Serve with lemon wedges for squeezing, and an apple and watercress salad on the side.

calories 336.50 ▪ fat 17.93 ▪ protein 34.33 ▪ carbohydrates 12.0

Marinated tuna steak
with mushroom
and parsley salad

Fresh tuna is increasingly easy to buy and it is a delicious fish, especially when marinated as it is here. This is another dish that you can prepare in advance: it only takes a very few minutes at the grill to finish it off.

Serves 2 ▪ Prep time: 30 minutes ▪ Cooking time: 10 minutes

2 x 100g tuna steaks
2 tbsp lime juice
1 tbsp olive oil
200g thinly sliced button
  mushrooms
100g flat leaved parsley, finely
  chopped
juice of two lemons
sea salt and black pepper

Place the tuna steaks in a bowl with the lime juice and half of the olive oil. Turn them so that they are coated and set them aside for at least half an hour.

Mix the mushroom slices, parsley, lemon juice, the remaining olive oil, salt and pepper, and cover with cling film. Set aside for the flavours to mingle.

When you are ready to eat, preheat the grill to high. Grill the tuna steaks for 5 minutes on each side, pouring any marinade over them as you turn them over. Serve with the mushroom salad.

calories 224 ▪ fat 8.47 ▪ protein 27.98 ▪ carbohydrates 11.75

Baked trout with flaked almonds and watercress salad

Trout and flaked almonds is a traditional combination of flavours, and the colours look magnificent on the plate.

Serves 2 ▪ Prep time: 5 minutes ▪ Cooking time: 25 minutes

2 trout, gutted but unwashed (the newspaper sticks better this way)

2 sheets tabloid-sized newspaper

120g bag watercress, or rocket/spinach/watercress salad

20g butter

2 tbsp olive oil

30g flaked almonds

1 juicy lemon

sea salt and black pepper to taste

Preheat the oven to 180°C/350°F/Gas Mark 4. Tip each trout onto a sheet of newspaper and wrap it up into a neat parcel, tucking the edges underneath. Place the parcels on a baking tray and bake for 25 minutes (or 20 minutes, if the trout are quite small).

While the trout are cooking, wash the watercress and place it in a salad bowl. When the trout are almost done, melt the oil and butter in a heavy-based saucepan and fry the almonds until they are a golden brown. Remove the almonds from the oil (keep the oil) and toss them with the green salad, adding the juice of half the lemon, a pinch of salt and a few grindings of pepper.

When the trout are done, peel away the newspaper carefully (the trout skin sticks to it) to leave a perfectly skinned trout on each plate. Pour the oil from frying the almonds over the trout, then slice the rest of the lemon thinly and arrange the slices decoratively. Serve with the almond-speckled green salad on the side.

calories 344 ▪ fat 4.08 ▪ protein 8.88 ▪ carbohydrates 32.60

Lentil salad
with lardons

Another simple, nourishing and tasty lunchtime meal, which you could eat with toasted pitta bread or a wholemeal roll.

Serves 1 ▪ Prep time: 2 minutes ▪ Cooking time: 6 minutes

50g lardons or cubed pancetta

100g cherry tomatoes

1 x 125g tin Puy lentils,
  drained

1 tbsp finely chopped parsley

1 tbsp balsamic vinegar

Grill the lardons or pancetta until crisp, then drain on kitchen paper and set aside.

Halve the cherry tomatoes, and mix with the lentils, parsley and vinegar. Put onto a serving plate and top with the lardons.

calories 245 ▪ fat 2.61 ▪ protein 22.43 ▪ carbohydrates 33.62

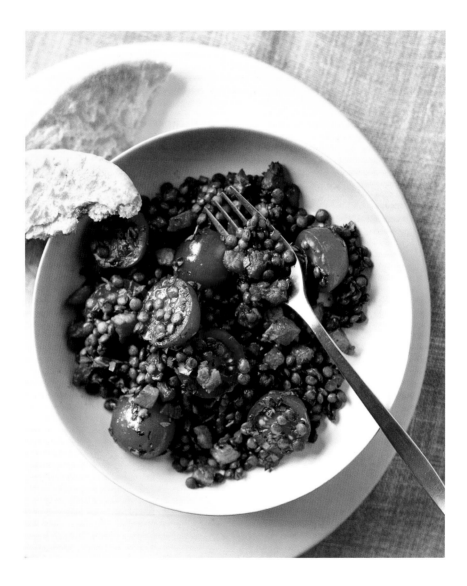

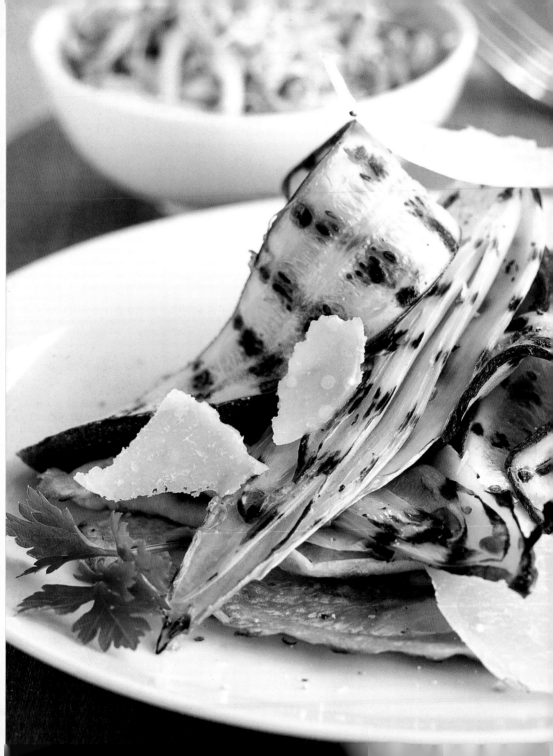

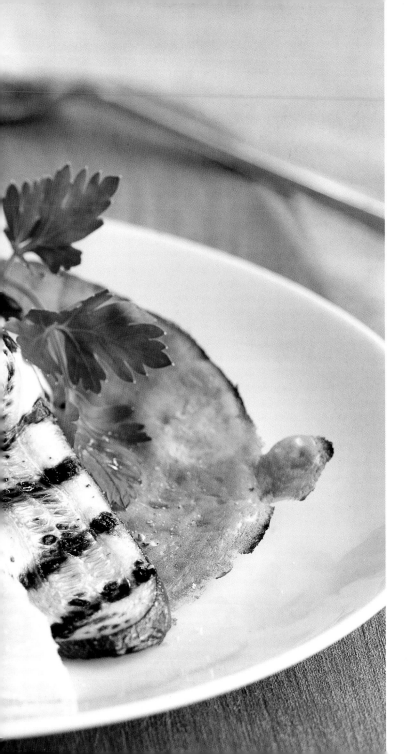

dinners

Thai green curry

You can buy ready-made green curry sauce, but it is so much nicer when it is fresh. This may look complicated, but if you prepare all the ingredients beforehand it is actually extremely easy and is well worth the effort.

Serves 4 ▪ Prep time: 5 minutes ▪ Cooking time: 15 minutes

1 x 410g tin low-fat coconut milk

3 tbsp Thai green curry paste

200g lean beef or chicken breast, thinly sliced

1 medium aubergine, cut into 2cm pieces

50g green beans, topped and tailed

1 x 410g tin baby corn, drained

1 x 410g tin of mushrooms, drained

2 tbsp brown sugar

2 tbsp fish sauce

3 kaffir lime leaves, stem removed and thinly sliced (or use 2 tbsp lime juice with the zest of ½ lime)

60g fresh basil leaves (set a few aside for garnish)

2 large, long chillies (1 red and 1 green for colour), sliced lengthways (to garnish)

FOR THE ACCOMPANYING VEGETABLES

2 tsp vegetable oil (not olive oil)

2 x 100g packs of mixed vegetables for stir-fry

In a wok, stir-fry the coconut milk for 5 minutes over a high heat. Add the green curry paste and continue to stir-fry for another 2 minutes. Add the chicken or beef pieces and cook for a minute, just until they begin to change colour. Add the aubergine pieces and continue to cook until they are just soft.

Now add the green beans and cook for another 2 minutes before adding the tinned mushrooms and baby corn.

Add the brown sugar and stir to dissolve, then add the fish sauce, kaffir lime leaves (or lime juice and zest), and basil.

Pour into a serving dish, quickly rinse out the wok and return it to a high heat with a teaspoon of vegetable oil.

Tip the vegetables into the wok and stir-fry briskly for a minute or so until they are just cooked but still retain some crunch.

Garnish the curry with some basil leaves and the sliced red and green chillies.

calories 457.5 ▪ at 26.66 ▪ protein 24.31 ▪ carbohydrates 38.84

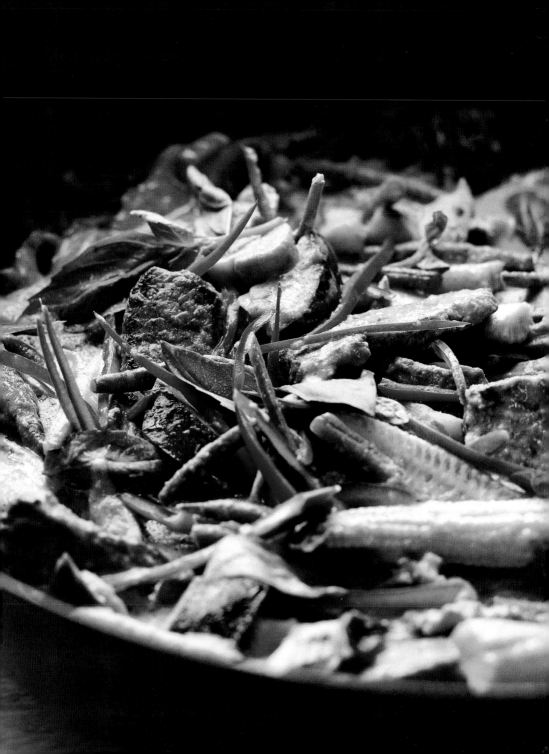

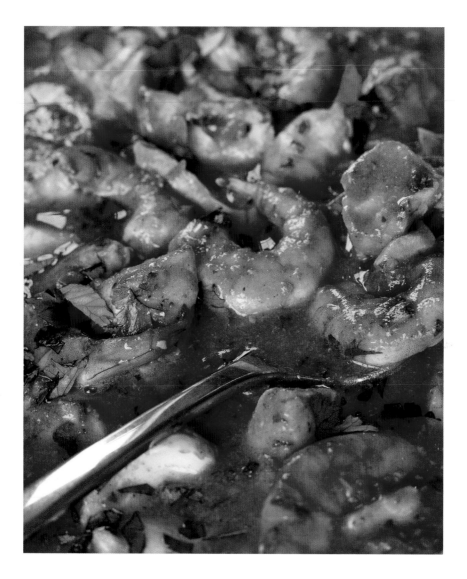

Easy fish and prawn curry

This is an unbelievably easy way of cooking fish, but extremely tasty. It's great to throw together when you get home: it'll be ready by the time you've wound down from your day. If you are using frozen fish or prawns, make sure that they are thoroughly defrosted before you begin.

Serves 2 ▪ Prep time: 5 minutes ▪ Cooking time: 30 minutes

2 x 100g fillets skinless white fish, such as haddock, coley or cod

100g prawns

1 x 410g tin chopped tomatoes in tomato juice (tinned cherry tomatoes work very well)

125ml semi-skimmed milk

2 tbsp flour

1 tbsp curry paste

50g fresh coriander, chopped

Preheat the oven to 180°C/350°F/Gas Mark 4. Chop the fish into bite-sized chunks, mix with the prawns and place in a shallow baking dish.

Put the chopped tomatoes, milk, flour and curry paste into a bowl and stir well with a wooden spoon until there are no floury lumps at all.

Stir in half the chopped fresh coriander, then pour the tomato mixture over the fish and prawns. Cover the dish with tinfoil and bake for 30 minutes. Sprinkle over the rest of the fresh coriander before serving. This goes very well with peas or green beans.

calories 259.50 ▪ fat 2.58 ▪ protein 33.17 ▪ carbohydrates 27.5

Chicken fillet
en papillote

Cooking 'en papillote' (in an envelope) is a lovely way to keep the moistness and flavour in. It's particularly good for chicken.

Serves 2 ▪ Prep time: 10 minutes ▪ Cooking time: 30 minutes

2 x 100g chicken fillets
2 bay leaves
peppercorns
2 tbsp white wine
2 large tomatoes
2 tsp olive oil
a sprinkle of thyme leaves or dried thyme
200g runner beans, topped, tailed and chopped

Preheat the oven to 180°C/350°F/Gas Mark 4.
Put each chicken fillet on a square of tin foil, place a bayleaf and a few peppercorns on top of each one, and drizzle the wine over them. Form a sealed parcel by folding the tinfoil loosely around the chicken and crimping the edges together. Place in an ovenproof dish.

Cut the tomatoes in half, across their width. Sprinkle them with the thyme, a pinch of salt, a few grindings of pepper, and a drizzle of olive oil. Place the tomatoes in another ovenproof dish and bake them, with the chicken, for 30 minutes.

Bring a pan of salted water to the boil. Simmer the beans for 5 minutes, drain and serve with the chicken and baked tomatoes.

calories 316.50 ▪ fat 7.87 ▪ protein 40.13 ▪ carbohydrates 21.01

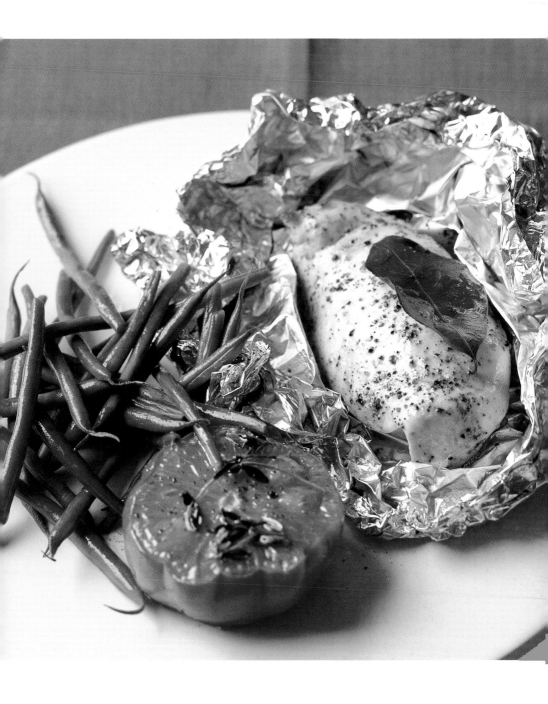

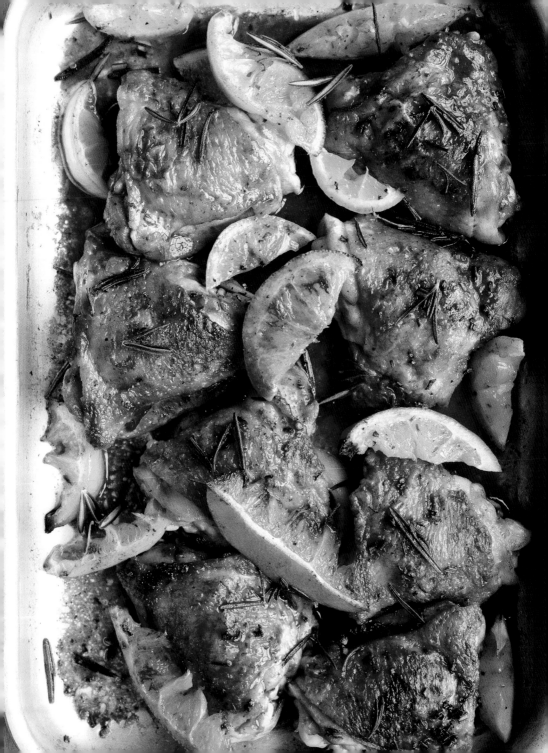

Tray-baked citrus chicken with lentils and rocket

This is great for a dinner party as there is so little to do, but it has so much flavour and it also looks tasty.

Serves 6 ▪ Prep time: 5 minutes ▪ Cooking time: 45 minutes

8 chicken thighs

1 unwaxed lemon, cut into quarters

2 oranges, cut into quarters

125ml chicken stock (fresh, if you can find it)

2 tbsp balsamic vinegar

4 sprigs rosemary

½ tsp sea salt

a few grindings of black pepper

2 x 410g tins of cooked lentils, drained

2 x 100g bags rocket, or spinach/rocket/watercress salad

1 tbsp olive oil

Preheat the oven to 180°C/350°F/Gas Mark 4. Squeeze some of the lemons and oranges into a small bowl. Add the stock and balsamic vinegar, season, and mix well.

Cut each citrus piece in half again. Arrange the chicken in a large baking dish, tucking the orange, half of the lemon pieces, and three rosemary sprigs in between the thighs. Pour over the stock mixture, cover with tin foil and place in the centre of the oven for 20 minutes. Remove the foil, baste the chicken pieces; then turn the heat up to 200°C/390°F/Gas Mark 6 and cook for another 20 minutes to brown the chicken.

When the chicken is done, turn off the oven, remove the chicken and gently squash the citrus pieces to release a little more juice. Carefully pour or ladle all the juices into a saucepan. Re-cover the chicken with the tinfoil and leave it to rest in the oven with the door ajar.

Boil the chicken juices vigorously for a few minutes, then tip the lentils into the pan with the remaining rosemary, season and warm them through. Serve with the green salad, dressed with a little olive oil and the juice squeezed from the reserved lemon pieces.

calories 350.33 ▪ fat 10.55 ▪ protein 31.69 ▪ carbohydrates 33.49

Roasted autumn veg
with soy-marinated tofu

This colourful mix is full of vitamins and anti-oxidant properties. Tofu is also one of the best sources of plant hormones and provides essential fatty acids.

Serves 2 ▪ **Prep time: 15 minutes** ▪ **Cooking time: 30–40 minutes**

4 beetroot, cooked, peeled and quartered

1 medium-sized butternut squash, chopped into fairly large chunks

2 fennel bulbs, trimmed, halved and par-boiled

a bunch of young carrots, cut into strips

1 large red onion, cut into 6 wedges

2 cloves of garlic, unpeeled

3 tbsp olive oil, or use olive oil spray

sea salt and freshly ground black pepper

1 tbsp herbed or spiced ground flaxseed seasoning (optional)

FOR THE TOFU

125g plain tofu, cut into bite-sized cubes

2–3 tbsp soy sauce

hot chilli sauce (optional)

TO FINISH

a good handful of chopped parsley or coriander

dish of pickled chillies

low-fat yoghurt, cream cheese or yofu alternative, for dolloping

wedges of lemon, for squeezing

Preheat the oven to 200°C/400°F/Gas Mark 6. Spray a roasting tin with olive oil to cover. While the oven is heating up, you can par-boil the firmer vegetables for 3 minutes if you don't want them too crunchy.

Spray all the vegetables with olive oil or toss in 2–3 tablespoons of olive oil. Season well and then wedge in the unpeeled cloves of garlic. Roast for 30–40 minutes, turning the vegetables once during cooking. If they need a bit longer, turn the oven down to a medium heat and cook for a further 10 to 15 minutes.

While the vegetables are roasting, marinate the tofu cubes in a spoonful or two of soy sauce for at least half an hour – a bit longer won't hurt. Heat up a wok or frying pan, spray with oil and sauté the tofu, tossing repeatedly until it begins to get crispy in places – then dash in a drop more soy, or a splash of hot chilli sauce.

Dish the roasted vegetables onto warmed plates. Squeeze the sweet garlic purée from the skins into the hot pan to mix with the tofu and then tip over the vegetables. Sprinkle with lots of chopped herbs and serve immediately with the pickled chillies, yoghurt and lemon wedges.

calories 209.5 ▪ fat 5.61 ▪ protein 8.57 ▪ carbohydrates 34.41

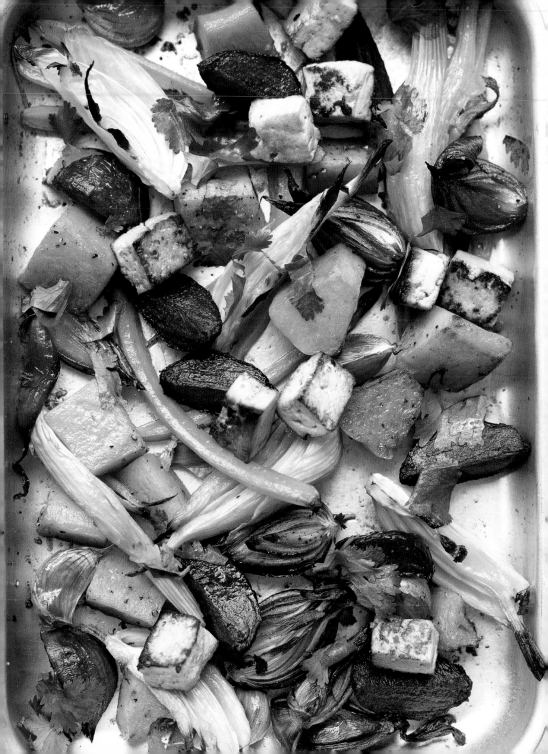

Teriyaki chicken on red onion and mushrooms

Teriyaki sauce is traditionally used in Japanese cooking to give a dark glaze to meat or vegetables. It is easy to make yourself and keeps for weeks in the cupboard. It goes extraordinarily well with mushrooms and the leftover sauce can be used to flavour soups or stir-fries.

Serves 2 ▪ Prep time: 10 minutes ▪ Cooking time: 25 minutes

TO MAKE YOUR OWN
TERIYAKI SAUCE:

150ml dark soy sauce

100ml rice mirin

1 tbsp dark muscovado sugar

FOR THE CHICKEN

1 tbsp olive oil

1 red onion, halved and thinly sliced

250g flat cap or Portobello mushrooms, cleaned and sliced (about 1cm thick)

2 pieces of tinfoil, about 30 x 20cm

2 x 100g skinless chicken breasts

2 tsp teriyaki sauce (see above)

100g Savoy cabbage leaves, washed, trimmed and cut into chunky pieces

To make the teriyaki sauce, place all the ingredients in a heavy-bottomed saucepan and bring to the boil, stirring gently to dissolve the sugar. Turn the heat down and simmer for about 10 minutes, until the liquid has reduced by half. Cool, and store in a clean jam jar.

Preheat the oven to 200°C/390°F/Gas Mark 6. Heat the olive oil in a non-stick frying pan over medium heat. Add the red onion and sliced mushrooms, and fry until the mushrooms turn dark brown. Divide the mixture evenly between the two pieces of tinfoil, and place a chicken breast on top of each one.

Rub a teaspoon of teriyaki sauce over each chicken breast, then make a parcel out of the tinfoil. Don't wrap it tightly or the foil will stick to the chicken; but do make the parcel as airtight as possible so that the steam can't escape. Place the parcels on a baking tray and place in the oven for 20 minutes.

When the chicken is done, take it out of the oven and leave it to stand while you cook the cabbage in boiling water. Drain the cabbage, divide it between the plates and then, opening the parcels carefully, tip the chicken, mushrooms and all the glorious juices over the top.

calories 317 ▪ fat 10.73 ▪ protein 35.78 ▪ carbohydrates 18.32

Asian-flavoured chowder

A traditional chowder is a soup made with milk; here I use silken tofu to give the same creaminess, but without the fat. You can find silken tofu in health food shops; it is very versatile, absorbs flavours without changing them, and is full of goodness. Add some to your morning smoothie for an early protein hit.

Serves 4 ▪ **Prep time: none** ▪ **Cooking time: 15 minutes**

300ml vegetable stock (use fresh stock, not a stock cube)

600ml water

1 tsp ginger purée

½ tsp sea salt

300g canned sweetcorn, drained

200g silken tofu

juice of half a lime

½ tsp toasted sesame oil

2 spring onions (green and white parts), thinly sliced

Put the stock, water, ginger purée, salt and two-thirds of the sweetcorn into a pan. Bring to the boil and simmer gently for 10 minutes.

Remove from the heat, add the silken tofu and blend until fairly smooth. Add the rest of the sweetcorn and simmer for another 3 minutes. Add the lime juice, stir it in and check for salt and to see if you need to add more lime juice.

Ladle into bowls, then sprinkle a few drops of sesame oil and the spring onions on top.

calories 108 ▪ fat 3.22 ▪ protein 5.29 ▪ carbohydrates 17.39

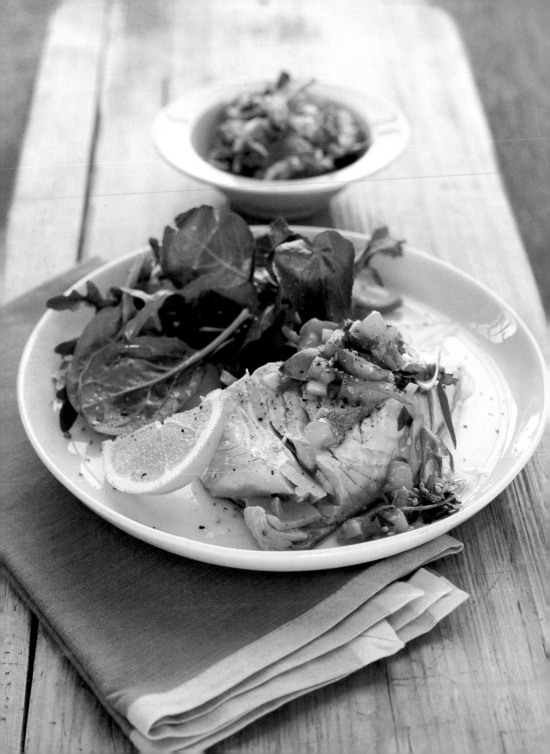

Aromatic summer salmon with purple grape and mango salsa

Steaming is an easy and healthy way to cook fish as it preserves the essential Omega 3 fats and makes for a very light and fresh-tasting meal. The red grapes will rebuild strength for tomorrow's workout!

serves 2 ▪ prep time: 10 minutes ▪ cooking time: 15 minutes

FOR THE FISH

2 x 100g fillets salmon

sea salt and freshly ground black pepper

1 lemon

2 spring onions

a few shavings ginger

FOR THE SALSA

1 bunch spring onion, trimmed but including some of the green part

1 clove garlic, peeled and finely chopped

1 tbsp ginger, grated

1 mango, cubed

1 nectarine, cubed (optional) small bunch purple grapes, halved

1 handful coriander, chopped

1 handful mint, chopped mixed flax and sesame seeds, toasted

2 tbsp red grape juice

generous squeeze lemon juice

SERVE WITH

salad mix of baby spinach, rocket and watercress

Set up the steamer and put the water on to boil. Mix all the salsa ingredients together in a bowl, season to taste and then set aside for the flavours to develop while the salmon is cooking.

Rinse the salmon under cold running water and pat dry with kitchen paper. Season the fish with a little sea salt, freshly ground black pepper and a good squeeze of lemon juice.

On two sheets of lightly oiled kitchen foil, make a bed of spring onion and ginger and lay the salmon on top with a squeeze of lemon. Loosely crimp and seal the foil and then place both parcels in the steamer tray. Steam for approximately 15 minutes.

Arrange the salad leaves on two plates. Heap a good serving of the salsa in the middle and top with the hot, steamed aromatic salmon.

calories 292.5 ▪ fat 7.32 ▪ protein 22.17 ▪ carbohydrates 37.54

Mexican vegetable soup

This is extremely easy to make, freezes well, and has a lovely smoky flavour. The refried beans add both protein and thickening to the soup; if you can't find them, then use an extra can of pinto or cannellini beans instead, mashing them up with a fork before you put them into the pot. Eat the soup as soon as possible after it's prepared, so that you don't lose the vibrant green colour of the French beans. If you like your soup hot and spicy, you can use bottled salsa, but I prefer it with the fresh tomato taste.

Serves 4 ▪ Prep time: 10 minutes ▪ Cooking time: 15 minutes

1 tsp olive oil

1 medium red onion, finely chopped

2 cloves garlic, finely chopped

½ tsp ground coriander

2 medium carrots, peeled and cut into bite-sized chunks

1.25 litres vegetable stock (or 1.25 litres water and two vegetable stock cubes)

1 x 415g tin refried beans

1 x 415g tin cannellini beans

½ tsp dried oregano

1 tbsp chopped jalapeno chillies (from a jar)

350g green French beans, topped, tailed and cut into bite-sized chunks

juice of ½ a lime

FOR THE TOMATO SALSA

2 medium tomatoes,

1 spring onion, thinly sliced

30g (a small bunch) fresh coriander, finely chopped

juice of ½ a lime

½ tsp salt

Mix together the ingredients for the salsa and set aside.

Use a heavy-bottomed pan to fry the onions in the oil over a medium heat. When they are translucent, add the garlic and ground coriander and fry for a minute more. Add the carrots, vegetable stock, refried beans, cannellini beans and dried oregano and bring gently to the boil, stirring fairly regularly. Simmer for 5 minutes, then add the jalapeno chillies, French beans and lime juice. Simmer for another 3 minutes, check for salt and then serve, putting a good dollop of the tomato salsa in the middle of each bowl.

If you want to freeze the leftovers, add any remaining salsa to the soup beforehand and as you reheat the soup you can refresh the taste with a little more lime juice and chopped fresh coriander.

calories 248 ▪ fat 3.22 ▪ protein 13.24 ▪ carbohydrates 44.4

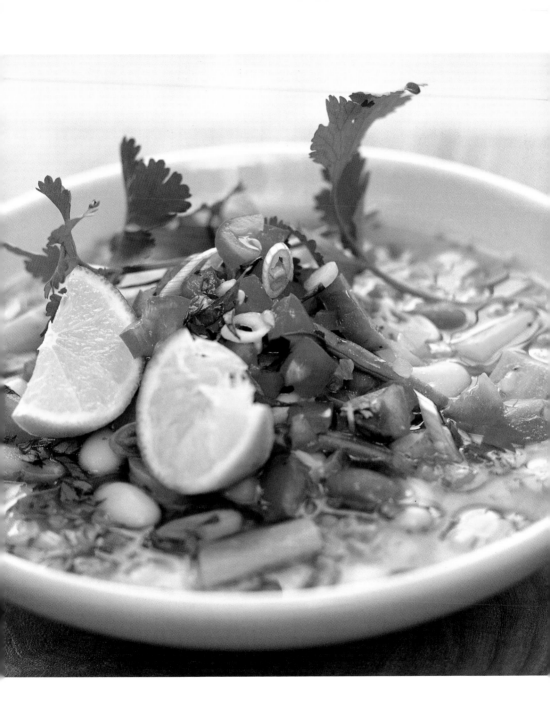

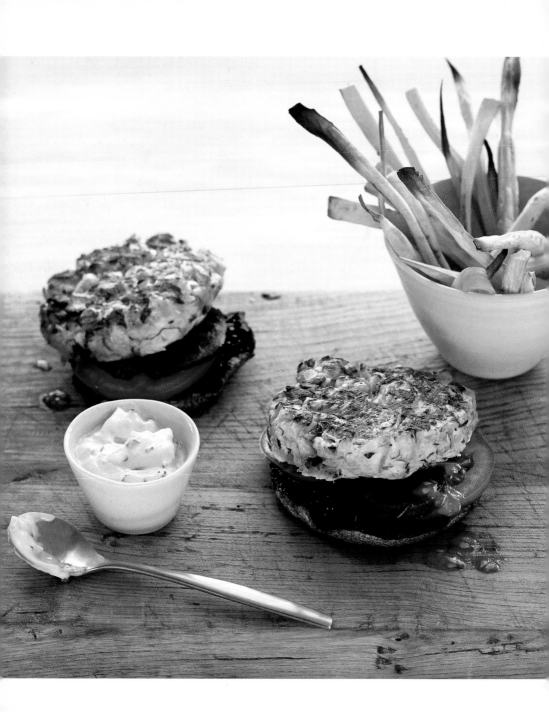

Chilli chicken and white bean burgers

Flaxseed (linseed) is an abundant source of Omega 3 and Omega 6 essential fatty acids, has a pleasant nutty flavour and will reduce and even replace the need for salt. Serve these flaxseed-enriched burgers my Carb Curfew way, balanced on a large, baked field mushroom 'bap' with parsnip chips on the side.

Serves 2 ▪ **Prep time: 15 minutes** ▪ **Cooking time: 40 minutes**

FOR THE BURGERS

200g drained (canned) canellini beans

200g skinless chicken breast, minced or roughly chopped

75g grated courgette

75g grated carrot

4 spring onions, sliced

2 cloves garlic, finely chopped

1 red chilli, finely chopped

1 tablespoon ground flaxseed good handful coriander, chopped

3 teaspoons olive oil

Sea salt and freshly ground black pepper

1 small egg, beaten

TO SERVE

3 medium parsnips, peeled and sliced into chip wedges

2 large field mushrooms

3 beef tomatoes, sliced

3 beetroots, sliced

FOR THE SOYA 'MAYO'

5 chopped radishes

3 tbsp yofu/low fat natural yoghurt

Preheat the oven to 200°C/400°F/Gas Mark 6 and lightly spray a baking tray with olive oil. At the same time, line a roasting tray with tin foil and set aside. Spray the parsnips with a little olive oil and roast in the oven for 40 minutes, turning occasionally.

Mash the drained beans roughly and then purée half of them to a smooth texture. In a large bowl, combine the beans with the chicken, courgette, carrot, spring onions, garlic, chilli, flaxseed, coriander, olive oil and seasoning, using your hands to thoroughly mix together. Carefully add just enough beaten egg so that the mixture holds together, without being too soft.

Divide the burger mix into 4 pattie shapes and place on the baking tray. Bake in the oven for about 30 minutes, without turning them. Halfway through cooking, drizzle a teaspoon of olive oil on top of each mushroom and add them to the tray.

Mix the radishes with 3 tablespoons yofu and season to taste. Balance each burger on a large mushroom and spoon over the soy 'mayo' to taste. Serve with a tomato and beetroot salad.

calories 434.5 ▪ fat 11.4 ▪ protein 40.08 ▪ carbohydrates 45.18

Gammon steak with Puy lentils and stir-fried greens

Lentils have an undeservedly bad reputation: they are delicious if properly cooked and served with complementary flavours. The orange juice in this dish gives it a real lift, and goes very well with the stir-fried greens. If you're not familiar with Puy lentils, they are small, very dark green and don't need presoaking.

Serves 2 ▪ Prep time: 5 minutes ▪ Cooking time: 20 minutes

200g Puy lentils

2 bay leaves

2 x 100g gammon steaks

juice of two oranges (blood oranges, if you can find them)

400g Savoy cabbage leaves, shredded and rinsed

2 tbsp soy sauce

Preheat the oven to 180°C/350°F/Gas Mark 4. Cover the lentils generously with water, add the bay leaves and bring to the boil. Simmer gently for 20 minutes.

Put the gammon steaks side by side in an ovenproof dish. Pour the orange juice over them and cover lightly with tin foil. Put in the oven and bake for 10 minutes.

While the lentils and gammon are cooking, stir-fry the cabbage with a few drops of water for a few minutes until it begins to wilt, then add the soy sauce and put the lid on. Allow to steam for a further 5–10 minutes, stirring occasionally.

Serve the gammon on a bed of lentils with the cooking juice poured on top, and the cabbage on the side.

calories 363.5 ▪ fat 7.86 ▪ protein 31.54 ▪ carbohydrates 47.39

Chickpea and almond crêpes

These high-protein, low-fat crêpes (see page 74) are highly versatile and can be used as a base for all manner of Carb Curfew, low-calorie suppers.

Recipe illustrated on page 74

Serves 2 ▪ **Prep time: 5 minutes** ▪ **Cooking time: 5 minutes**

FOR THE CRÊPES
110g almonds, ground
50g chickpea flour
1 tbsp flaxseed
1 egg
200ml soya milk
a pinch of sea salt
olive oil spray
water, if necessary

FOR THE TOPPING
2–3 medium courgettes (200g)
1 head chicory
garlic and herb flavoured
   olive oil
handful of parsley, chopped
handful chives, snipped
a little Parmesan, grated

TO SERVE
1 small pack mixed
   beansprouts

Blend all the crêpe ingredients until smooth and set aside while you prepare the vegetables. Warm a plate for stacking the pancakes in a medium oven.

Preheat the griddle pan so that it is hot. Wipe the courgettes with dampened kitchen paper and slice lengthways into long strips, not more than 0.5cm thick. Break off leaves of chicory. Spray them with olive oil, season lightly and place on the hot griddle pan, turning from time to time until they are slightly charred.

While the vegetables are grilling, take the crêpe mix and if necessary add water to thin it slightly. Spray a non-stick pan with olive oil and heat to medium/hot. Pour in 1 ladle of the mixture and swirl it round the pan so that it covers the base. After about 30 seconds, the edges will begin to set. When you see this, flip the crêpe over and cook for 30 seconds on the other side. Transfer to a warmed plate and cover while you cook the next ones.

To serve, dish 1 or 2 pancakes onto each plate and top with the chargrilled vegetables, some flavoured oil and a little grated Parmesan. Shower with lots of chopped parsley and chives and a beansprout salad on the side.

calories 422.5 ▪ fat 28.07 ▪ protein 20.49 ▪ carbohydrates 28.5

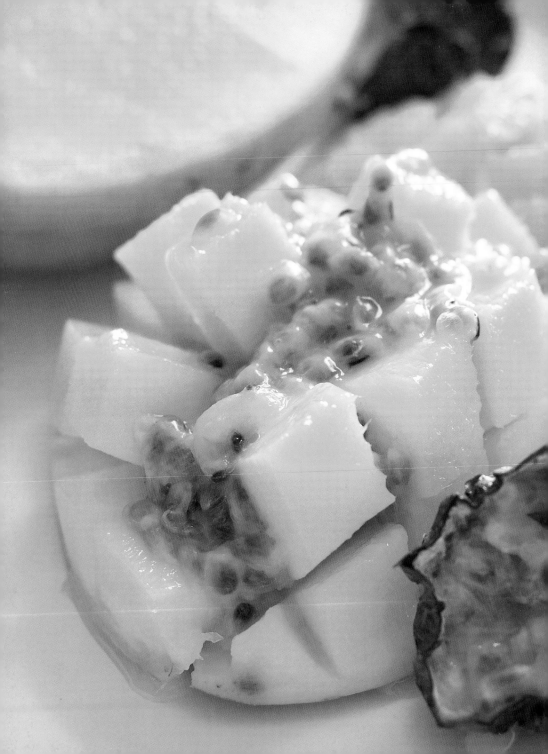

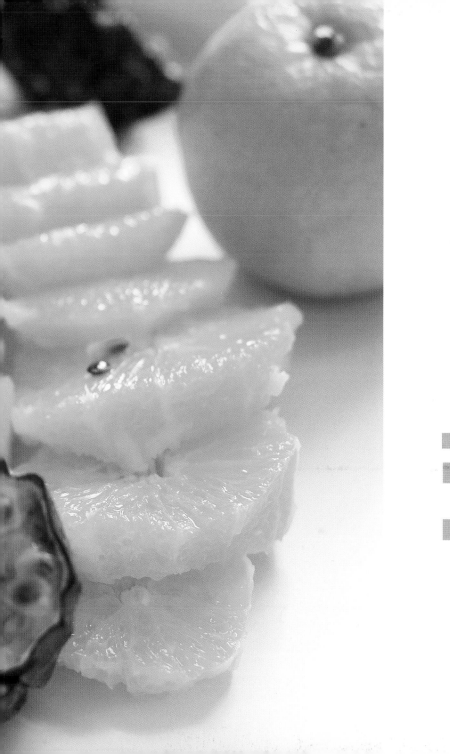

puddings

Orange, mango and passion fruit

Recipe illustrated on page 96

Passion fruit give a great deal of taste for their size. Look for the purple ones that have gone all wrinkly on the outside, as they are likely to be the sweetest.

Serves 4 ▪ Prep time: 20 minutes ▪ Cooking time: 5 minutes

3 passion fruit
2 tsp honey
6 juicy sweet oranges
1 large or 2 small mangoes, good and ripe
zest of 3 of the oranges, cut into very fine strips

Cut the tops off the passion fruit and scoop out the insides with a teaspoon, putting them into a small saucepan.

Add the honey and 2 tablespoons of water, and heat gently until the orange flesh has dissolved and the black pips are floating freely (you don't have to do this, but it stops the passion fruit clumping together). Leave to cool.

Peel the oranges and cut off as much of the pith as you can. Use a serrated knife to cut them into thin rings then lay them in a serving dish. Cut the stone out of the mango, and peel and roughly chop the flesh. Mix this with the oranges and pour over the passion fruit – pips and syrup.

Sprinkle the orange zest over the top and leave in the fridge for several hours if you can, for the flavours to develop.

This is best served chilled but not straight from the fridge (coldness tends to kill the flavours).

calories 123.75 ▪ fat 0.37 ▪ protein 2.12 ▪ carbohydrates 31.56

Rhubarb and strawberry jelly

Experiment with different fruit for this easy, make-in-advance dessert. You could try fresh blueberries in a lemon jelly, poached apricots in raspberry jelly... the combinations are endless. Serve in Martini glasses, or large wine goblets, to show off the gorgeous colours.

Serves 4 ▪ **Prep time: 15 minutes** ▪ **Cooking time: 15 minutes**
Setting time: 6–8 hours

200g rhubarb
1 tbsp lemon juice
1 packet sugar-free
   strawberry jelly

Wash and slice the rhubarb into 1cm lengths. Place them in a covered saucepan with the lemon juice and cook over a gentle heat for 5–10 minutes, stirring occasionally. Strain the rhubarb, reserving the juice.

Make up the jelly, as per packet instructions, incorporating the rhubarb liquid in the required amount of water. Leave to cool to room temperature before carefully mixing in the cooked rhubarb, and pouring into the serving dishes.

Leave to set in the fridge for at least 6 hours.

calories 11.25 ▪ fat 0.11 ▪ protein 0.47 ▪ carbohydrates 2.52

Baked bananas
en papillote

A grown-up version of banana splits, warm and spicy.

Serves 4 ▪ **Prep time: 5 minutes** ▪ **Cooking time: 20 minutes**

4 bananas
juice of 2 oranges
2 tsp grated orange rind
2 tsp grated lemon rind
a few pinches of cinnamon
125g low-fat natural yoghurt
50g toasted slivered almonds
(optional)

Preheat the oven to 180°C/350°F/Gas Mark 4. Place each banana in a square of foil large enough to fold up into a little tent. Add the orange juice, orange and lemon rind and cinnamon and seal each parcel with a double fold. Place the tents on a baking tray and bake for 20 minutes.

You can just lift the tents onto the plates and let everyone unwrap them. Serve natural yoghurt and toasted slivered almonds on the side.

without almonds
calories 65.0 ▪ fat 0.68 ▪ protein 2.19 ▪ carbohydrates 13.51

with almonds
calories 111.75 ▪ fat 4.78 ▪ protein 3.92 ▪ carbohydrates 15.11

Cinnamon-poached fruit

This works well as a cold dessert, but is also great in the morning with a dollop of low-fat yoghurt. It keeps for days in the fridge if you cover it with cling film. Choose your own combination of fruit, or buy 'dried fruit salad' from the health food shop.

Serves 6 ▪ Prep time: 5 minutes ▪ Cooking time: 40 minutes

250g mixed dried apple, apricot, pineapple, prunes, mango, cherry, blueberry

2 cinnamon sticks

4 tbsp honey

Place the dried fruit in a large heavy-based casserole dish with the cinnamon sticks and honey. Pour in water to cover it by at least 2cm and simmer gently for 40 minutes, checking frequently to make sure that the water hasn't evaporated: you want a good amount of delicious juice to serve with it.

When the fruit pieces have plumped and softened, remove from the heat, leave to cool and then refrigerate. This dish benefits from being made the day in advance to allow the flavours to develop. Depending on your choice of fruit, you may want to add a little more honey before serving.

calories 143.83 ▪ fat 0.21 ▪ protein 1.07 ▪ carbohydrates 38.23

Peaches baked with mascarpone

Another very easy dessert. Use fresh peaches in season (wait until they are fully ripe or they tend to be tasteless) or you can use tinned peaches for this dish.

Serves 4 ▪ Prep time: 5 minutes ▪ Cooking time: 20 minutes

2 peaches
4 tsp mascarpone cheese
2 tsp granulated sugar
20g toasted almond slivers

Preheat the oven to 180°C/350°F/Gas Mark 4. Halve and stone the peaches and place them in an ovenproof dish, cut side up. Place a teaspoon of cheese in the hollow of each peach half, and sprinkle with half a teaspoon of sugar.

Cover the dish loosely with tin foil and bake for 10 minutes. Remove the tin foil and bake for another 10 minutes. Sprinkle the toasted almond slivers over each peach, and serve.

calories 51.0 ▪ fat 1.67 ▪ protein 1.75 ▪ carbohydrates 7.92

Chocolate chip banana cake

Who says you can't have chocolate cake when you're trying to lose weight? Here's a recipe for a delicious treat that's not too high in calories – because you're worth it!

Serves 8 ▪ Prep time: 10 minutes ▪ Cooking time: 25 minutes

125g butter
60g granulated sugar
60g brown sugar
2 medium eggs
2 small ripe bananas
250g flour
½ tsp salt
½ tsp baking soda
4 tbsp plain yoghurt or sour cream
1 tsp vanilla extract
185g chocolate chips
½ tsp cinnamon mixed with a little caster sugar

Preheat the oven to 180°C/350°F/Gas Mark 4, and grease and flour a 23 x 30cm baking tin. Cream the butter and sugar together until the mixture is light and fluffy (approximately 5 minutes with electric stand mixer). Add the eggs, one at a time, beating well after each addition and then the bananas, mixing well and scraping the sides.

Sift the dry ingredients together, and then add them to the butter and sugar mixture. Add the yoghurt (or sour cream) and vanilla, followed by the chocolate chips and mix together well to obtain a smooth batter, but do not overbeat.

Pour the batter into your prepared tin, and liberally sprinkle cinnamon-sugar mixture over the top of the cake. Bake for approximately 25 minutes on the middle shelf of the oven. When the cake's ready a skewer will come out clean.

calories 432 ▪ fat 18.24 ▪ protein 7.05 ▪ carbohydrates 63.5

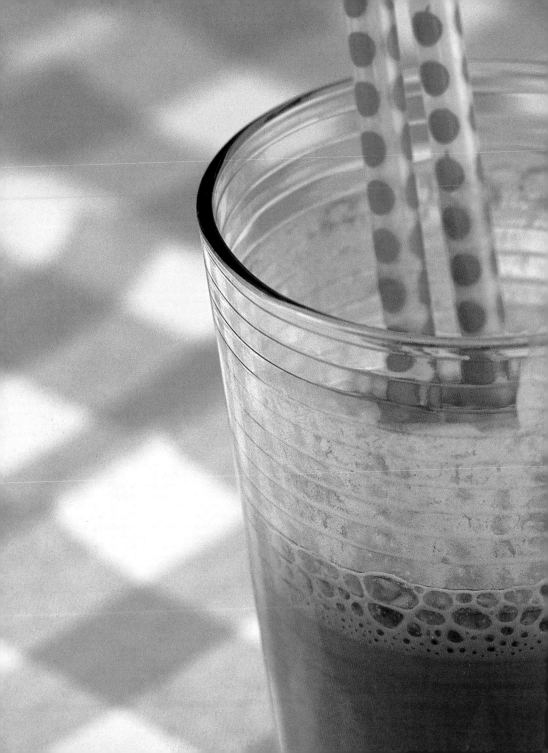

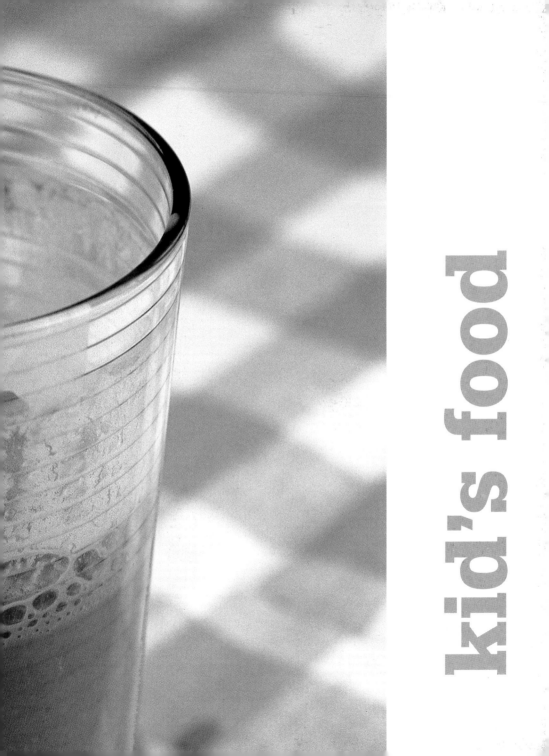

kid's food

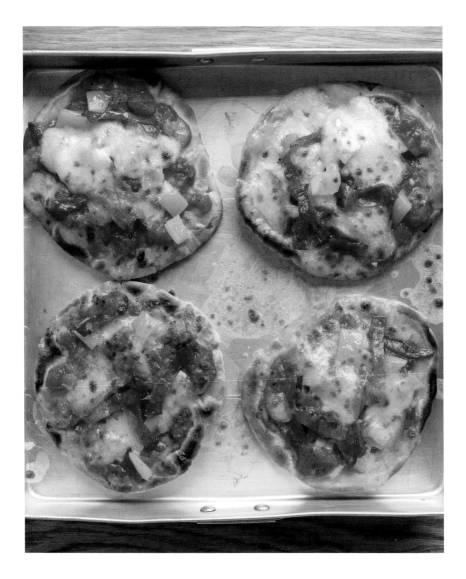

Pitta bread pizzas

This is the really easy way to make pizzas, and it's fun for kids because they can choose and arrange their own toppings. There is very little fat if you make them this way, and you can keep pitta breads on hand in the freezer. To make pizzas from frozen pitta bread, increase the cooking time by 2 minutes.

Serves 4 ▪ **Prep time: 5–10 minutes** ▪ **Cooking time: 8 minutes**

1 x 410g tin chopped tomatoes

1 tsp dried mixed herbs (or ½ tsp each of thyme and oregano)

8 regular or 4 large white pitta breads

TOPPINGS:

Choose from olives, thinly sliced red or green peppers, a couple of rounds of salami cut into thin strips, wafer thin ham, small chunks of canned pineapple. For more adult tastes, try a few thin slices of aubergine, some sliced mushrooms, anchovies, or a teaspoon of pesto sauce.

200g grated low-fat mozzarella cheese

Preheat the oven to 230°C/450°F/Gas Mark 6. Mix the herbs with the chopped tomatoes in a small bowl, and then spread thinly on each of the pitta breads. Add a selection of toppings, then sprinkle the grated mozzarella over the top.

Bake for 8 minutes or until the cheese is golden brown. It's as simple as that!

calories 319 ▪ fat 8.84 ▪ protein 18.4 ▪ carbohydrates 41.27

Healthy chicken nuggets with easy baked chips

If only all chicken nuggets were made this way... And if only all chips actually tasted of the potatoes they are made of, instead of the fat they're fried in.

Serves 4 ▪ Prep time: 15 minutes ▪ Cooking time: 30 minutes

FOR THE NUGGETS

2 x 200g chicken breasts, skin removed and chopped into bite-sized chunks

4 tbsp plain flour

2 large eggs, beaten with 2 tbsp water

2 Weetabix, crumbled fine, or 6 tbsp dry breadcrumbs

6 tbsp vegetable oil

¼ tsp paprika

a pinch of salt

few grindings black pepper

FOR THE CHIPS

4 x 200g large roasting potatoes, cut into thin wedge shapes

2 tbsp vegetable oil

a pinch of salt

Preheat the oven to 200°C/400°F/Gas Mark 6. Spray the potatoes with the vegetable oil and lightly sprinkle a little salt on them. Arrange the potato wedges on one end of the baking tray, and cook for 15 minutes.

While the chips are cooking, set up your production line: you will want a plastic bag with no holes in it, three bowls and a piece of baking parchment. Have the bowl with the egg and water mix on the left (or right, if you're left-handed), then the bowl with the breadcrumbs or crumbled Weetabix, then the bowl with the vegetable oil, then a piece of baking parchment. Put the flour and the chicken chunks into the plastic bag, and shake vigorously until all the chicken is well coated. Place this bag on the far side of the bowl with the water and egg mixture.

Take a floured chicken chunk, roll it quickly in the egg mix, then in the Weetabix crumbs until it's well coated, then spray it with the oil, and place it on the baking parchment. Repeat with the rest of the chunks.

After the chips have had 15 minutes in the oven, remove the baking tray and flip the chips over with a spatula. Add the chicken nuggets to the tray and return to the oven for 15 minutes until everything is golden brown.

calories 475 ▪ fat 29 ▪ protein 22.31 ▪ carbohydrates 31.17

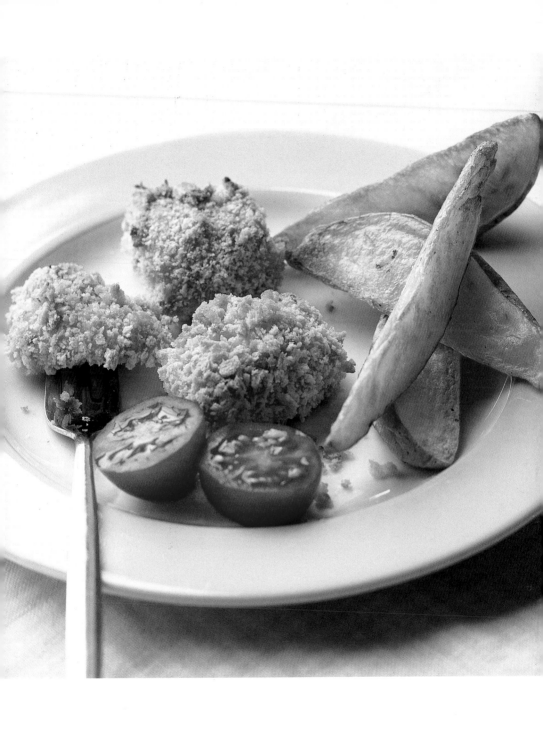

Banana-chocolate smoothie

Recipe illustrated on page 104

A delicious way to start the day – and a great means of getting breakfast into children.

Serves 2 ▪ Prep time: 3 minutes ▪ Cooking time: none

150g low-fat bio live yoghurt

300ml semi-skimmed milk

2 heaped tsp drinking chocolate

2 ripe bananas, sliced, or 100g fruit (see below)

ALTERNATIVES ARE:

100g strawberries and 2 tsp drinking chocolate

100g raspberries and 2 tsp drinking chocolate

1 ripe mango and a few sprigs of fresh mint to decorate

100g stewed apricots and some chopped lemon zest

Put the yoghurt, milk, drinking chocolate and banana (or fruit) into a blender. Whizz on high speed for 30 seconds, until smooth.

Play around with the fruit combinations.

calories 191.50 ▪ fat 4.08 ▪ protein 8.88 ▪ carbohydrates 32.60

eat yourself thin

Banana-sour cherry bread

This is very good toasted for breakfast or between-meal snacks. A tasty treat that's healthy as well!

Serves 6–8 ▪ **Prep time: 10 minutes** ▪ **Cooking time: 1 hour**

225g plain flour
1 tsp salt
1 heaped tsp baking powder
1 tsp ground cinnamon
110g caster sugar
1 egg, beaten
90g unsalted butter, melted
a few drops vanilla essence
90g dried sour cherries
3 very ripe bananas, mashed

Preheat the oven to 180°C/350°F/Gas Mark 4. Sift together the flour, salt, baking powder and cinnamon. Stir in the sugar. With a fork, mix in the egg, melted butter and vanilla essence. Add the mashed bananas and cherries and mix with a fork just until all the ingredients are incorporated: don't overmix.

Spoon the mixture into the prepared tin and bake for 50–60 minutes until the loaf springs back when prodded. Leave in the tin for 10 minutes before turning it out to cool.

calories 282.38 ▪ fat 10.32 ▪ protein 3.67 ▪ carbohydrates 45.18

Index

Activity chart, 16
Alcohol, 39, 40
Aromatic summer salmon
    with purple grape and
    mango salsa, 89
Asian-flavoured chowder, 87

Balanced diet, 20
Bananas
    baked en papillote, 100
    banana muffins, 52
    banana-chocolate
        smoothie, 110
    banana-sour cherry
        bread, 111
    chocolate chip banana
        cake, 103

Calories, 16, 17
Carb curfew, 20, 21, 36
Carbohydrates, 21
Chicken
    Caesar salad with Cajun
        grilled chicken, 65
    chicken fillet en papillote,
        80
    chilli chicken and white
        bean burgers, 93
    healthy chicken nuggets
        with easy baked ships,
        108
    teriyaki chicken on red
        onion and mushrooms, 86
    tray-baked citrus chicken
        with lentils and rocket, 83
Chickpea and almond crepes,
    95
Chocolate chip banana cake,
    103
Cinnamon-poached fruit, 101
Curry
    fish and prawn curry, 79
    Thai green curry, 76

Date and pumpkin-seed loaf,
    51
Dietary fibre, 26

Egg, poached on Marmite
    toast with orange juice, 54
Energy gap, 16

Fad diets, 10, 11
Fats, 23, 24
    lowering intake of, 37
Food combining, 10, 11
Food IQ test, 12-15
Food labels, 33

Gammon steak with puy lentils
    and stir-fried greens, 94
Glycaemic index, 22

Healthy eating, 26, 32, 33
    children, for, 44, 45
Herring, grilled on oatmeal, 67
High-protein, low carb diet, 11

Juicing, 27
Junk food, 44

Lentil salad with lardons, 70
Liquid-based foods, 39

Mackerel, Italian-style, 62
Menu plans, 41–43
Mexican vegetable soup, 90
Minerals, 27, 31
Moosewood sesame citrus
    delight, 54

Nutrients, 20

Omega 3 and 6 fats, 23, 24
Orange, mango and passion
    fruit, 98

Peaches baked with
    mascarpone, 102
Pinhead oatmeal porridge
    with raisins, 50
Pitta bread pizzas, 107
Portion distortion, 37, 38
Proteins, 25, 37

Rhubarb and strawberry jelly,
    99
Roasted autumn veg with
    soy-marinated tofu, 84

Salt and sodium, 29
Spicy fruity coleslaw with
    ham, in pitta bread, 61
Sugarbusters and cravers, 11

Teriyaki tofu with red peppers
    and houmous roll-up, 64
Trout, baked with flaked
    almonds and watercress
    salad, 69
Tuna
    marinated tuna steak with
        mushroom and parsley
        salad, 68
    tuna, mushroom, parsley
        and lemon stuffed pitta, 60

Vitamins, 27, 30

Water, 28

Yoghurt
    blueberry-yoghurt slush
        with granola, 55
    natural, with granola and
        apple puree, 55

Zone diet, 11